A HANDBOOK OF SKIN DISEASES

A HANDBOOK OF SKIN DISEASES:

AND THEIR HOMEOPATHIC TREATMENT

JOHN R. KIPPAX

GYAN

Published by

GYAN

Gyan Publishing House
5, Ansari Road
Daryaganj, New Delhi-110002
Phone: 011-47034999, 9811692060
E-mail: books@gyanbooks.com

Distribution Network
gyanbooks.com
India, USA, Canada, UK, Australia

ISBN: 978-93-7133-771-7 (HB)

First Published, 1884

2nd Impression 2025

Printed at: Gyan Press, Delhi.

A HANDBOOK OF SKIN DISEASES
Author: JOHN R. KIPPAX

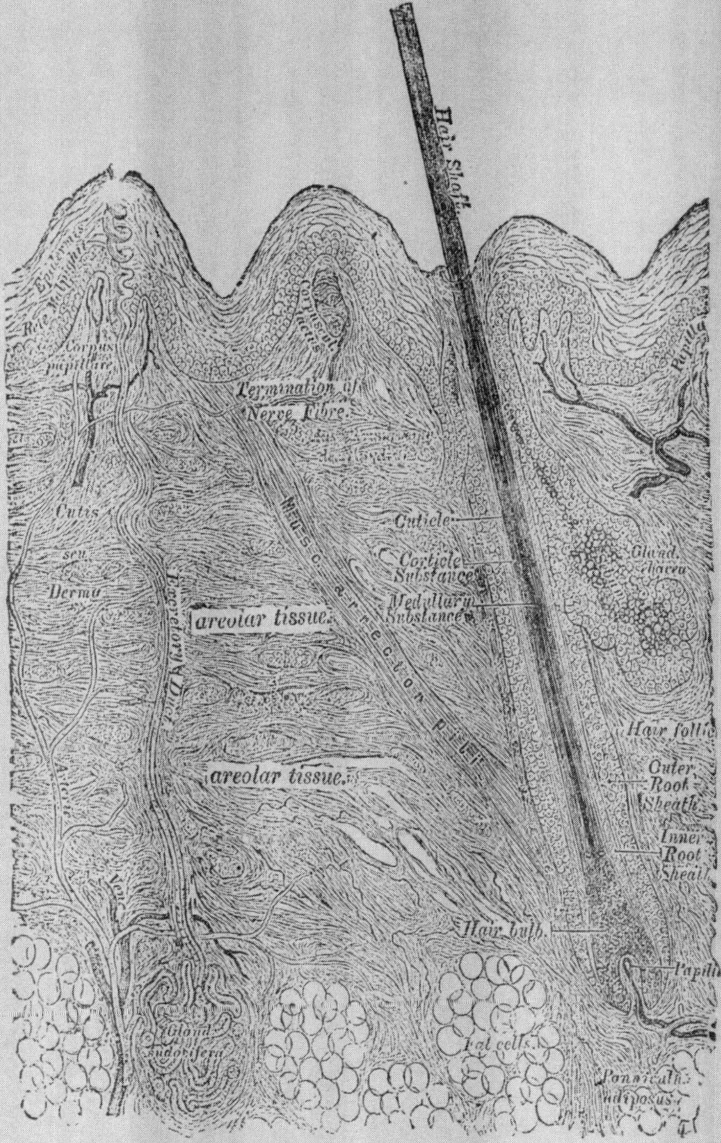

GENERAL VIEW OF THE SKIN AND ITS APPENDAGES (after Heitzmann).

A HAND-BOOK OF SKIN DISEASES, AND THEIR HOMŒOPATHIC TREATMENT.

BY

JOHN R. KIPPAX, M. D., LL. B.,

PROFESSOR OF PRINCIPLES AND PRACTICE OF MEDICINE AND MEDICAL JURISPRUDENCE IN THE CHICAGO HOMŒOPATHIC MEDICAL COLLEGE; LATE CLINICAL LECTURER AND VISITING PHYSICIAN TO COOK COUNTY HOSPITAL; MEMBER OF THE AMERICAN INSTITUTE OF HOMŒOPATHY; MEMBER OF THE COLLEGE OF PHYSICIANS AND SURGEONS, ONTARIO; AUTHOR OF LECTURES ON FEVERS, ETC, ETC.

1884.

To

ALL PRACTITIONERS

AND

STUDENTS OF HOMŒOPATHY,

TRUSTING IT WILL MEET

THEIR APPROVAL,

THIS VOLUME

IS RESPECTFULLY DEDICATED.

PREFACE TO THE SECOND EDITION.

In preparing this edition for the press, the entire text has been thoroughly and carefully revised. Owing to the unprecedentedly rapid advance in dermatological science, many portions of the book have been entirely re-written, and much new matter has been added.

It is hoped that the work, as revised, will merit a continuance of the favorable recognition extended to the previous edition by the profession.

J. R. KIPPAX.

CHICAGO, November, 1883.

PREFACE TO THE FIRST EDITION.

The design of the present Hand-book is to furnish such a digest of the essentials of practical dermatology, as will be serviceable alike to students and practitioners. In preparing the manuscript I have steadily kept one purpose in view, to make it as thorough and practical as possible. To this end condensation has been more or less necessary, and if at times statements appear too absolute, it must be remembered that conciseness and the limits of the book, prevented any lengthy discussion.

The text consists of short general observations on the anatomy, physiology, and pathology of the skin, and on the symptomatology, etiology, diagnosis and classification of cutaneous diseases; followed by a detailed description of each individual affection, giving its clinical history and treatment. To this is added a chart, with diagnostic, therapeutic and dietetic hints, which it is believed will be found extremely useful.

Another feature in the work is the pronunciation of the various medical words used, and the introduction of definitions.

* * * * * * * * * *

In regard to nomenclature, I believe matters have been simplified very materially, although originality is by no means claimed for the classification presented.

This Hand-book is virtually condensed from notes originally intended for a larger work, and is the result of careful study of the literature referred to in the Bibliography, combined with extensive clinical experience. Every effort, within the limits assigned in the original plan, has been made to lay before the profession a satisfactory compendium of dermatology in its present stage.

* * * * * * *

With these prefatory remarks I give this work to the profession, trusting it may, to a certain extent at least, supply the present want for a concise and practical exposition of cutaneous affections and their homœopathic treatment.

CHICAGO, May, 1880.

CONTENTS.

PART FIRST.

PART SECOND.

PART THIRD.

PART FOURTH.

PART FIFTH.

PART SIXTH.

DISEASES OF THE SKIN.

PART I.

GENERAL OBSERVATIONS.

SECTION I. THE ANATOMY AND PATHOLOGY OF THE SKIN.

The skin is a flexible membrane which invests the body, and joins the mucous surfaces at the various orifices. Its office is to protect the underlying structures from harm, to give shape and symmetry to the human form, to act as a partial respirator, and to perform the important functions of secretion, absorption, and tactile perception. Upon its surface are found numerous elevations, furrows and depressions. The larger elevations, which take the form of lines or wrinkles, are particularly well defined on the palm of the hand and sole of the foot. The smaller elevations are found upon almost all regions of the body, and are caused by the prominence of the papillæ. The furrows correspond to the larger elevations and lie between them. The minute depressions or pores, are the orifices of glandular ducts and of hair-follicles.

Like most tissues of the body the skin is composed of fibres and cells.

The fibres are of two kinds: white fibrous tissue, and yellow elastic fibres. The white fibres give to the skin strength, and the yellow, elasticity.

The cells are of four kinds, namely, the cells of the rete or stratum malpighii; secondly, those of the stratum granulosum; thirdly, those of the stratum lucidum; and fourthly, those of the stratum corneum.

The cells of the stratum malpighii are nucleated, polygonal in form, and rich in protoplasm. When isolated they resemble in outline a chestnut burr, and hence are termed "prickle cells."

The cells of the stratum granulosum are spindle-shaped, have a distinct, clear nucleus, and are arranged in two rows.

Those of the stratum lucidum are flattened, indistinctly striated, and contain a staff-shaped, or flattened nucleus. They are formed from the cells of the stratum granulosum, and are arranged in three rows.

And lastly, those of the stratum corneum, or horny epidermis, are flattened, have no nucleus, and are usually larger than the other cells.

These six elements, the two kinds of fibres, and the four sorts of cells, constitute the main part of the structure of the skin.

Anatomically, the skin may be divided into two main layers, termed respectively the *corium* and *epidermis*. And again, these two may be subdivided; the former, into the reticular and papillary layers, and the latter into the rete malpighii, the stratum granulosum, the stratum lucidum, and the stratum corneum or horny layer.

The corium constitutes the larger part of the skin, and is made up by the interlacement of elastic fibres and connective tissue. It contains as organs peculiar to the skin, prominently, sebaceous and sweat glands. At the deepest part of this structure, masses of fat globules are found packed between the fibres of connective tissue, constituting the *panniculus adiposus*, or adipose tissue.

The external surface of the corium presents elevations, or nipple-like prolongations, called papillæ. These are largest about the female nipple, and corona glandis, and smallest over the general cutaneous surface. They present an average of 60,000 to the square inch and are the seat of the tactile corpuscles of Meissner. According to their internal structure they may be divided into two kinds, *vascular* and *nervous*.

The reticular layer is looser in texture than the papillary layer; and the inter-fascicular spaces are well marked.

An increase of the connective tissue elements is usually found in keloid, fibroma and scleroderma. And a fatty degeneration occasionally takes place in the new growth which destroys the connective tissue, as in xanthoma. The papillæ may at times become enlarged in psoriasis, and the reticular layer may become the seat of such parasites as the Guinea worm, the acarus scabiei and the pediculus.

Next to the papillary layer of the corium comes the stratum malpighii or rete. The cells of this structure are mainly polyhedral, excepting the lower rows which are fusiform and fill up the interpapular spaces to a level a short distance beyond the apices of the papillæ. The deeper layers of this stratum are the abiding places of cutaneous pigment.

A hyper-activity of rete cells exists in psoriasis, and epithelioma is supposed to take its departure from this membrane.

Beyond the stratum malpighii is the stratum granulosum, which consists of two layers of nucleated, spindle-shaped cells. It is best seen at the mouths of the hair follicles and near the nails.

The stratum lucidum follows it, and is made up of flattened transversely striated cells, arranged in three rows.

And after this comes the stratum corneum or horny epidermis. The deeper cells of the latter stratum are polygonal in shape, while the more superficial are flattened. Its cells are increased in amount in congested conditions of the skin, as in psoriasis; in inflammatory diseases, as in eczema and dermatitis exfoliativa; and in general hyperplasia, as in elephantiasis. They may be congenitally increased as in ichthyosis, or become hypertrophied as in callositas.

The cell layers of both the stratum corneum, the stratum lucidum, and the stratum granulosum, may be elevated along with portions of the rete, by fluid forcing its way up from beneath; and thus they form the walls of vesicles as in eczema or herpes on the one hand, or those of bullæ, as in pemphigus on the other.

The organs of the skin are: blood vessels, lymphatics, muscular fibres, and nerves, sweat glands, sebaceous glands, and hair follicles; the appendages are, the hair and nails.

The large trunks of both arteries and veins are situated in the deeper parts of the subcutaneous tissue, and after supplying the organs form a deep plexus in the deep layers of the corium. Branches from this plexus, ascend to just beneath the papillary layer of the corium, where they form a superficial plexus.

A hyperplasia of these vessels exists in telangiectasis. The superficial plexus is mainly affected in psoriasis, lichen and prurigo. Both plexuses may be implicated in eczema.

The lymphatics also form plexuses, generally one beneath each plexus of blood vessels, and lymph spaces are usually present in the corium. They play an important part in morphœa and are increased, both as to size and number, in elephantiasis.

The lymphatic element is also apparent in the glandular swellings of prurigo, and in the enlarged glands at the back of the neck in eczema of the scalp in children.

The muscular fibres of the skin exist in two forms, striated and smooth. The former are found principally in the skin of the face. They arise from the deeper seated muscles, and pass upwards to terminate in the corium. The latter appear either as anastomosing plexuses running horizontally, as in the scrotum, or as fasciculi, as in connection with the glandular apparatus of the skin. Contractions of the little muscles formed by the aggregation of these fibres, causes the conditions known as *cutis anserina* or "goose-flesh."

Little muscles of the smooth or unstriped variety, called *erectores pili* (erectors of the hair), arise from the internal sheath of the hair follicles, pass obliquely upwards around the sebaceous glands, and terminate in the upper part of the corium. They are supposed to erect the hair and to favor the exit of sebum from the sebaceous glands.

The nerves of the skin are surface branches of the nerve trunks that accompany the larger blood vessels in the subcutaneous tissues. They are composed of both medullated and non-medullated fibres. The medullated fibres terminate as a rule in the Pacinian and tactile corpuscles; while the non-medullated fibres end as a sub-epithelial plexus in the upper layers of the corium and in the rete mucosum, from which filaments ascend between the epithelial cells towards the stratum lucidum.

The Pacinian corpuscles are small, ovoid bodies, found in the subcutaneous connective tissues, upon the nerves of cutaneous supply. They occur in various regions, but are most numerous in the volar side of the hand and foot.

The tactile or touch corpuscles, also called corpuscles of Meissner or Wagner, are oval bodies found mostly in the papillæ of the corium. They are most numerous upon the last phalanges of the fingers, where they are found in about one of four of the papillæ.

Vaso-motor and trophic nerves supplying the vascular, muscular and glandular systems, are also found in the skin.

The cutaneous nerves, in addition, give to the skin the sense of touch, and are intimately connected with the physiological and pathological changes going on around them. They undergo organic alterations in zoster, leprosy, dermatalgia, and telangiectasis.

The *sweat* or *sudoriparous glands* are small reddish-yellow bodies composed of convoluted tubules situated in the deep parts of the corium, or even in the subcutaneous adipose tissue. They open on the external surface by means of a narrow efferent duct, which presents an oblique valve-like aperture.

They are found in all parts of the body, but are most numerous on the palms and soles. According to careful computation there are between two and three millions of them in the human body, representing an average of eight miles of perspiratory tubing.

By evaporation they tend to regulate the temperature of the body, and ordinarily throw off between one and two pints of fluid daily. They also act as auxiliary to the kidneys, in throwing off excrementitious matters. The natural perspiration is generally acid in reaction, and is composed of nearly ninety-eight per cent of water and two per cent of solid, mostly organic, materials. It is normally alkaline in the axilla and between the fingers and toes, and after prolonged sweating. It may become variously colored, as in chromidrosis; or impregnated with organic matters, such as urea, albumen, sugar or bile.

The sweat glands may become functionally disordered, as in hyperidrosis. They may be primarily affected, as in dysidrosis, or secondarily disordered as in ichthyosis.

The *sebaceous* or *sebiparous glands* are small pyriform sacculated organs lodged in the substance of the corium. They are composed of a basement membrane externally, and secreting cells, or their products internally. They are furnished with excretory tubes which open usually in the hair follicles, but occasionally upon the cutaneous surface. Generally there are two to each hair, located on opposite sides; at times four or even eight may be found grouped around a single hair-sac. They are to be met with upon all portions of the body, except the palms, soles, dorsum of the third phalanges, and the glans penis. The largest are those of the eyelids, the nose, the lips, the labia externa and the scrotum. The secretion from these glands is of an oily nature, and is known as sebaceous matter or sebum. It contains about fifty per cent of fatty matter, and is perfectly fluid at the ordinary temperature of the body. The office of the sebum is to prevent too rapid evaporation, and to give softness and pliability to the skin and to the hair.

The sebaceous glands may be functionally disordered, as in seborrhœa on the one hand, or as in xeroderma on the other. They may be primarily affected, as in acne, or secondarily diseased, as in elephantiasis and leprosy.

The *hairs* are peculiar modifications of the epidermis, and consist of shafts and roots. They are of three classes: (1.) Long and soft hairs, as those of the scalp, pubes, and axillæ. (2.) Short hairs, soft as those of the eyebrows, or stiff as upon the lids. (3.) Fine downy hairs, found upon the face and body and called *lanugo*.

The total number of hairs on the scalp has been estimated at from ninety to one hundred and twenty thousand. The cortical portion of the shaft of the hair is made up of firmly adherent, flat horny cells, while the medullary substance consists of a mass of loosely packed epidermal elements. The difference in constitution of the cortex and medulla of the hair gives to the structure minuteness, strength and elasticity. A single hair has been known to support a weight of over two ounces; and it is so very elastic that it may stretch almost one-third of its length, yet return to its former measurements.

The color of the hair is mostly given to it by the pigment granules that are found stored in the horny and medullary portions.

The root presents a bulbous enlargement which is closely connected with the papilla, a vascular eminence situated at the base of a finger-of-glove depression in the epidermis and corium, called the hair follicle.

The rate of growth of the hair is about a half inch per month. Hairs grow by the multiplication and pushing outwards of the cells of the bulb lying next to the hair papilla. They may become either hypertrophied or atrophied, or even texturally changed.

The *hair follicle* is cylindrical in form and is always placed more or less obliquely in the skin. It consists of a body, neck and mouth. The latter is funnel shaped and opens directly upon the surface. The neck is the narrowest part of the tube and is located just below the level of the papillary layer; while the body, which constitutes the largest part, terminates in a bulbous extremity and contains the hair papilla and the hair bulb.

The follicle consists of two parts, an outer, the hair sac, and the inner, the root sheath.

The *hair sac* is made up of three layers, external, middle and internal.

The external layer is the thickest and most important, and is composed of connective tissue fibres which run parallel with the course of the hair, and join the fibres of the papillary layer of the corium. The middle layer is highly contractile and is made up of transverse connective tissue fibres, embedded in a homogeneous, slightly granular substance. The internal layer is a homogeneous transparent tissue, and is a direct continuation of the basement membrane of the corium.

The *hair papilla* protrudes into the cavity of the follicle, and consists of connective tissue derived from its middle layer, together with round nuclei and nucleated cells. It is about twice as long as it is broad, and contains arteries, veins and non-medullated nerve fibres. The constricted portion of the papilla is the neck and the thicker part the body.

The *root-sheath* consists of two layers: (1.) The external; (2) the internal. The *external root-sheath* is a continuation of the rete malpighii, which extends into the level of the papilla. It is thinnest at the neck of the follicle, and thickest at the bulb.

The internal *root-sheath* is made up of (*a.*) an *outer* or Henle's layer; and (*b.*) an *inner* or Huxley's layer. The outer layer is a thin, transparent membrane composed of oblong non-nucleated scales which run parallel with the shaft of the hair. It commences at the neck of the follicle and terminates at the bulb. The inner layer consists of flattened fusiform nucleated cells containing small refractive granules.

As a rule there is only one hair in each follicle, but occasionally two are found to occupy a follicle conjointly.

The *nails* are horny, elastic, concavo-convex, structures imbedded in the skin upon the dorsum of the distal phalanges. They are composed of altered cuticular cells derived from the various strata of the epidermis.

The posterior portion of the nail, situated beneath the skin, is called the *root;* and the anterior exposed portion is termed the *body*. The corium upon which the nail rests and to which it is firmly attached is known as the *bed* or *matrix*.

The whitish disk, situated just in front of the posterior groove and due to the diminished transparency of the tissues is called the *lunula*.

Nails grow from their roots as do hairs, and simply slide over the matrix. They grow more rapidly in summer than in winter, and in early age than in adult life. They may become structurally changed, as in onychia. Or they may be primarily affected, hypertrophied, as in onychauxis, or secondarily so, as in psoriasis, syphilis and ichthyosis. Or, again, the vegetable parasites may here take up their habitat, giving rise to the condition termed onycho-mycosis.

The *subcutaneous tissues* are made up of variously sized loose bundles of connective tissue, containing usually an abundance of fat. When the fat cells are arranged in groups to form lobules and lobes, the structure is then called *adiposé tissue* or *panniculus adiposus*.

SECTION II.

SYMPTOMATOLOGY.

The clinical signs, or symptoms, of disease may be either objective or subjective. Objective symptoms are those appearances which manifest themselves upon the surface, and are capable of ocular demonstration. Subjective symptoms relate solely to sensations which arise from within, and are cognizant only to the patient.

The objective symptoms of diseases of the skin embrace all the elementary cutaneous lesions, whose physical characters may be roughly outlined as follows:

MACULES, SPOTS OR STAINS, ARE CIRCUMSCRIBED DISCOLORATIONS OF SKIN..

They are usually of a reddish, yellowish, or brownish color; and may be either permanent or evanescent. Small dot-like purpuric macules are called *petechiæ.*

Macules may be either primary as in lentigo or secondary as in Addison's disease. Sometimes they are physiological in character, as in pregnancy. They are met with in chloasma, nævus, purpura, morphœa, and erythema.

PAPULES OR PIMPLES ARE SMALL ACUMINATED ELEVATIONS OF SKIN VARYING IN SIZE FROM A MILLET SEED TO A SPLIT PEA.

They may be either true or false, and are frequently attended with itching. They are seen in acne, eczema, scabies, lichen, prurigo and milium.

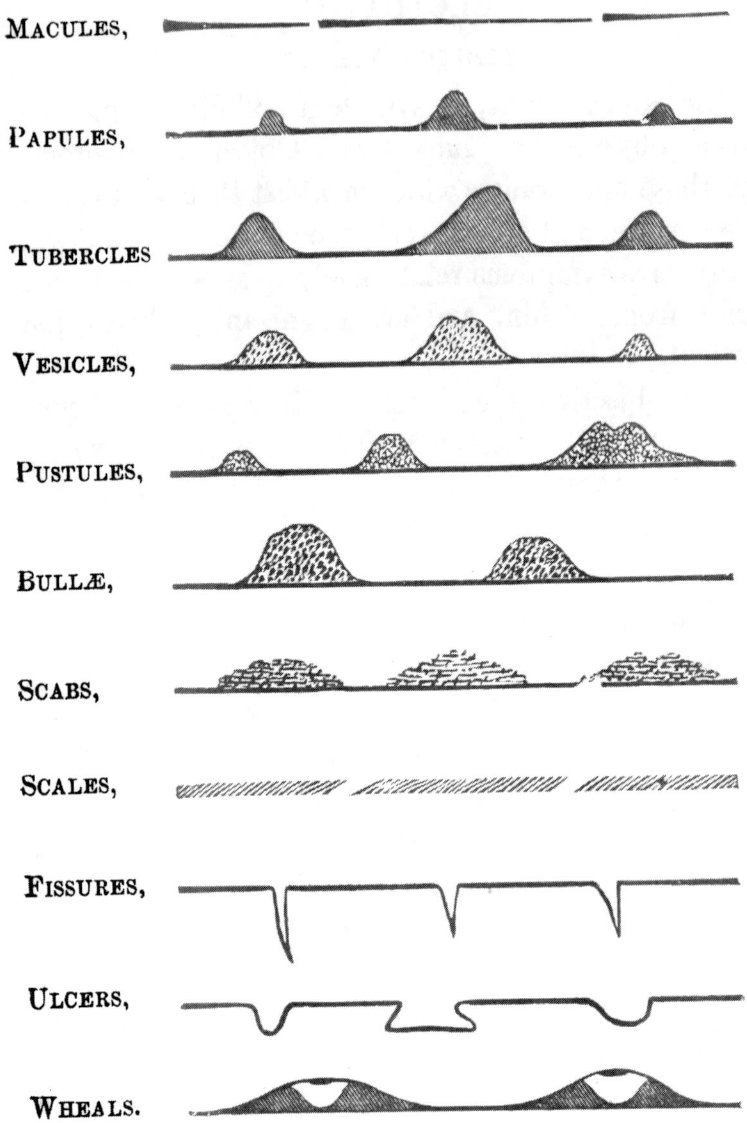

FIG. 2. Diagram of the principal elementary cutaneous lesions—in profile—(after Piffard).

Vesicles are small, elevations of the epidermis, enclosing a transparent or milky fluid, varying in size from a millet seed to a split pea.

They are as a rule inflammatory, and are usually accompanied by burning and itching. There are three kinds, viz.: serous, sweat and lymphatic. The serous are present in eczema, herpes, scabies, impetigo contagiosa and zoster. The sweat are seen in sudamina and dysidrosis. And the lymphatic are observed in elephantiasis.

Bullæ are blisters or large vesicles, varying in size from a split pea to a goose egg.

They occur in groups, and are not commonly attended by marked itching or burning. They may be either primary or secondary. They are primary in pemphigus, leprosy, and hydroa. And they are secondary or accidental in dysidrosis, eczema and urticaria.

Pustules are small collections of pus covered by epidermis.

They are of yellowish, yellowish-green, or brownish-green color, and are as a rule accompanied with areolæ. They may either originate as pustules, or become so by change from vesicles or papules. And they terminate either by rupture or by desiccation. They are met with in acne, eczema, impetigo contagiosa and ecthyma.

TUBERCLES ARE SMALL SOLID FLESHY SWELLINGS IN THE SKIN, VARYING IN SIZE FROM A SPLIT PEA TO A HAZEL NUT.

They are usually of a reddish color, and are commonly situated in the deeper layers of the corium or the subcutaneous connective tissue. They are seen in acne, tricophytina, sarcoma, fibroma, syphilis and leprosy.

WHEALS ARE RED OR WHITISH, TRANSITORY ELEVATIONS OF THE SKIN, RESEMBLING THE STING OF THE NETTLE, AND ACCOMPANIED BY TINGLING OR PRICKING SENSATIONS.

They are situated in the upper layers of the skin, and are produced by a rapid exudation and temporary incarceration of serum in the meshes of the corium, due to clonic vascular spasm. They are fugitive and capricious in character, and may appear either as elongated oval lines or stripes. They are pathognomonic of urticaria. Occasionally they result from insect bites and from medicinal poisoning.

SCALES, ARE COLLECTIONS OF ALTERED CELLS OF THE STRATUM CORNEUM.

They are usually whitish or yellowish in color, and have a shining or glistening aspect. They are observed in eczema, pityriasis, psoriasis, ichthyosis, seborrhœa, tricophytina, etc.

EXCORIATIONS, ARE SUPERFICIAL SOLUTIONS OF CONTINUITY OF THE SKIN.

They present a variety of forms, and as a rule, heal without leaving scars. They are observed in connection with eczema, scabies, phthiriasis; also in consequence of bites of insects; and in all disorders of the skin attended with pruritus.

FISSURES, ARE LINEAR SOLUTIONS OF CONTINUITY OF THE SKIN, SITUATED IN THE EPIDERMIS OR CORIUM.

They commonly appear about the normal furrows of the skin especially in the vicinity of the articulations, and are usually attended with pain. They occur in eczema, psoriasis, leprosy, and the syphilides.

CRUSTS, ARE FORMED BY THE DRYING UP OF DISCHARGES.

They are yellowish in color when formed by desiccation of serum; greenish-yellow when composed of dried pus; and brownish or blackish when they contain blood. They are found in eczema, ecthyma, impetigo contagiosa, leprosy, sycosis, seborrhœa, syphilis, etc.

ULCERS, ARE CIRCULAR SOLUTIONS OF CONTINUITY OF THE SKIN, USUALLY FOLLOWED BY CICATRICES.

They are most frequently met with on the lower extremities, and are usually attended with pain. They are the result of previous disease, and occur in lupus vulgaris, leprosy, scrofuloderma, furuncle, etc.

Scars or cicatrices, are new formations replacing lost tissue.

They are usually whitish in color, smooth, and somewhat depressed. They consist of connective tissue elements, and are devoid of hair follicles, papillæ or glands. They may follow ulcerative lesions, and are also seen in acne, favus, sycosis and zoster.

Of subjective symptoms, *sensations* of *heat, burning* and *tingling* are most common. They are met with in varied degrees in all hyperæmic and inflammatory cutaneous affections.

Pain is a general accompaniment of acute inflammation, as in zoster, etc.

Hyperæsthesia or over-sensitiveness of the skin is frequently met with in dermatalgia, and in the early stages of leprosy.

Anæsthesia or loss of sensibility is present in the later stages of leprosy, and in syphilis.

Pruritus or itching is one of the most prominent and annoying of the subjective symptoms. It may be due to local causes, or may be entirely dependent on reflex conditions.

SECTION III.

ETIOLOGY.

The etiology or causes of diseases of the skin may be conveniently considered under two heads: I. Internal or constitutional causes. II. External causes.

I. THE INTERNAL CAUSES which are also the most numerous, admit of arrangement and description as follows:

1. *Hereditability.*—An inheritable state in which diseases or taints may be handed down from parent to child. As striking examples, syphilis, leprosy, psoriasis, and ichthyosis, may be mentioned.

2. *Constitutional Tendencies.*—By which is to be understood a disposition either hereditary or acquired, to the developement of certain, usually inflammatory cases, under favorable conditions.

3. *Organic and Functional Diseases of the Internal Organs.*—Their name is legion. A few may be cited. Derangements of the alimentary canal, are frequent causes of cutaneous eruptions, notably of eczema, urticaria and acne. Uterine diseases may complicate or give rise to the same troubles. Disease of the kidney is a common cause, or aggravating condition in eczema. Derangement of the nervous system plays a prominent part in a variety of disorders. Venereal excesses lead to herpes, pruritus, and syphilis. And affections of the liver have considerable influence in shaping the course of a number of cutaneous ailments.

4. *Age* and *Sex* are important conditions influen-

cing disease. Certain affections are found to appear at stated periods of life, and are peculiar to one or the other sex. The congenital syphilide appears during the first months of infant life. Ichthyosis manifests itself in the second year. And impetigo contagiosa is in the majority of cases an affection of childhood. Of the parasitic affections, tricophytina, excepting when it attacks the beard, is more common in children, while tinea versicolor is oftenest met with in adults. Acne appears about the time of puberty. Epithelioma rarely shows itself before middle life, and is of more frequent occurrence in males; while lupus originates in childhood and is more common in females.

5. *Certain articles of food*, may, under peculiar conditions become essential factors in the causation of cutaneous eruptions. Of these should be noticed: shell-fish and strawberries as common causes of urticaria; cracked wheat, graham bread, oat meal and buckwheat, as giving rise to roughness of the skin and pruritus; stimulating drinks, preserved meats, and highly seasoned food, as aggravating influences in eczema, urticaria and acne.

6. *Drug Poisoning.*—The overdosing with such drugs as Mercury, the Potassium Bromide and Iodide, Quinine and Fowler's solution, Copaiba and Valerian, Chloral and Salicylate of Soda, is frequently productive, in Old School practice, of cutaneous complications. Notably may be mentioned the eczema mercuriale, the urticaria caused by Valerian and Copaiba, the

acne produced by the Potash salts, and the scarlatinal rash induced by Chloral and Salicylate of Soda.

II. THE EXTERNAL CAUSES, are:

1. *Climatic Influences.*—Some diseases are aggravated in, or peculiar to cold climates, while others flourish in tropical regions. The majority of cutaneous disorders are aggravated by cold weather. A few as for instance prickly heat, are peculiar to warm seasons. While certain diseases, such as leprosy, elephantiasis, and pellagra, are almost peculiar to certain countries. As a general rule in any locality, temperature will exert an influence, proportionate to the extremes of heat and cold to which the patient is subjected.

2. *Irritants.*—Want of cleanliness is the exciting cause of many skin affections. The tinea fungus riots in dirt, and filth is a condition favorable to the development of eczema and other cutaneous inflammations. Pruritus is frequently due to the frictional effect of clothing. Traumatism may give rise to excoriations and even infiltrations of the skin. Local irritants are often met with in particular occupations. Grocers, masons and bakers are often troubled with eczema, induced by handling flour or lime. Washerwomen, workers in dyes and the wearers of dyed garments, are also frequently the subjects of the same disease.

3. *Parasites.*—Of these there are many varieties, both animal and vegetable, each parasite producing its own characteristic contagious lesion, and only requiring a favorable soil on which to fructify and grow.

SECTION IV.

DIAGNOSIS.

The diagnosis of cutaneous affections is, to the experienced eye, an easier task than that of any other class of diseases. The predominance of objective symptoms which serve at all times as "key-notes," enables the physician with a little aid from the patient in the way of subjective symptoms, to ascertain positively the extent and nature of the lesion. The examination must in all cases be thoroughly instituted. The family history of the patient should be learned, and the occupation and habits inquired into. The physical characters of the eruption must be closely scrutinized, and the peculiar features of the extending edges of the patches accurately determined. To this end, it is necessary to examine all the affected portions of the skin, special attention being given to the newest developments. The changes, if any, in the character of the eruption from the time of its first appearance should be carefully noted, and the stages through which the disease has already passed, satisfactorily mapped out. It must be borne in mind that the influences of temperament, age, sex or social surroundings may modify the general characters and aspect of a disease; and that complications may so mask a case as to render it difficult of recognition.

The examination is best conducted in day light, admitted from a northern exposure. A white light is the best substitute for sunlight. In difficult or complex cases, where the unaided eye is unable to solve the problem, a microscope provided with a fifth and half inch objective, may be used with profit.

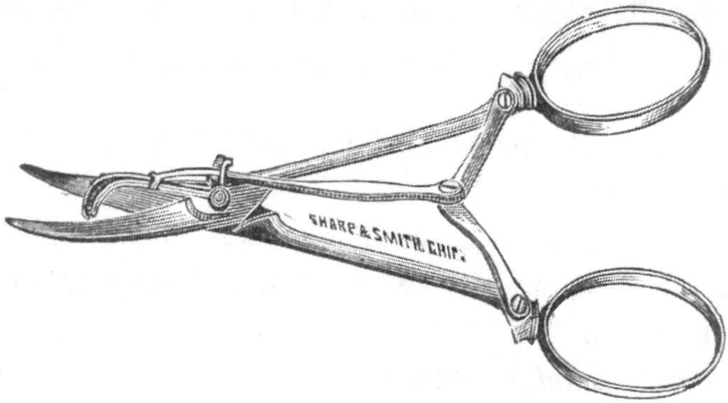

FIG. 3. SKIN-GRAFTING SCISSORS.

When necessary, as in affections of the beard or scalp, one or more hairs may be secured for examination by extraction with a pair of epilating forceps, (Fig. 12.) Small slices of other parts to be examined can be easily obtained by the use of the skin-grafting scissors, (Fig. 3.) or, if still thinner sections are needed, the cutisector (Fig. 4.) may be employed.

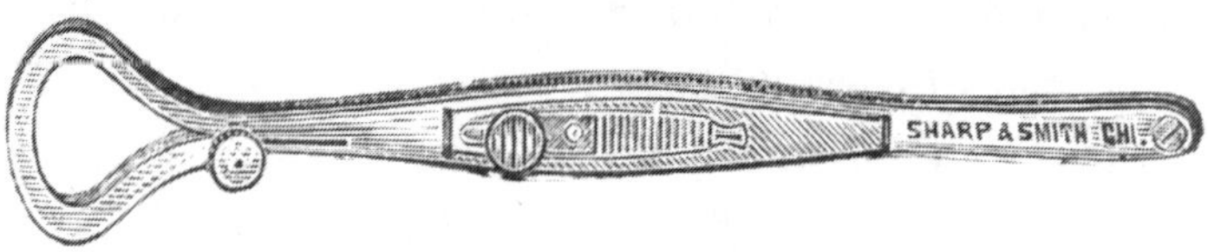

FIG. 4. THE CUTISECTOR.

The temperature of parts, if desired, is readily taken by Seguin's surface thermometer. (Fig. 5.)

Very material aid in making a diagnosis is frequently derived from remembering the locality

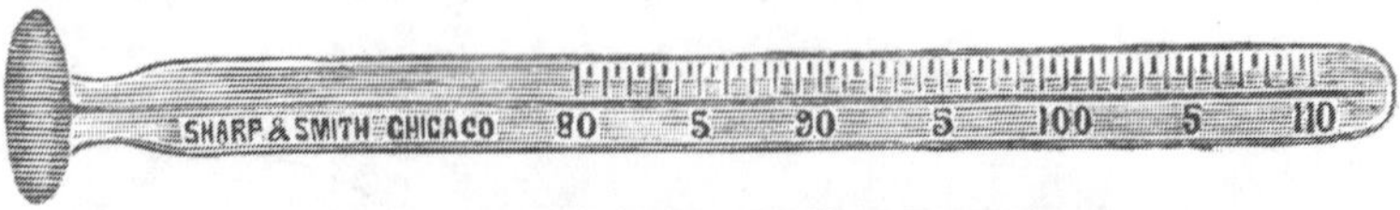

FIG. 5. SEGUIN'S SURFACE THERMOMETER.

attacked. The following table, after Fox, gives the main points:

The scalp, is the most common seat of seborrhœa, the tineæ, eczema, sebaceous cysts, psoriasis and alopecia areata.

The forehead, of acne.

The nose, of lupus and rosacea.

The cheeks, of lupus, rosacea and eczema.

The upper lip, of herpes and eczema.

The lower lip, of epithelioma.

The chin, of sycosis and tinea tricophytina.

The angle of the mouth, of epithelioma.

The ears, of eczema.

The front of chest, of kelôid and tinea versicolor.

Under the clavicle, of sudamina.

Region of the nipple, of scabies and Paget's disease.

The side of chest, of zoster.

The elbows and knees, of psoriasis.

The interdigits and front of wrists, of scabies.

Back of the hands, of lichen and eczema.

The palms, of syphilide.

The buttocks inner ankle and toes in children, of scabies.

The dorsum of penis, of scabies.

The scrotum, of eczema, psoriasis and chimney-sweepers' cancer.

The front of the leg, of dermatitis contusiformis.

The leg, if running around or lengthwise, of zoster.

The whole body, of pemphigus foliaceus and dermatitis exfoliativa.

And *the flexures of joints*, of eczema and scabies.

SECTION V.

CLASSIFICATION.

Classification is generally resorted to in order to simplify the study of disease, and is as important in the department of dermatology as in any other branch of medical science.

The arrangement here presented is a modification of that recently adopted by the American Dermatological Association.

CLASS I.

Disorders of the Glands.—(1.) Of the sweat glands: Anidrosis. Bromidrosis. Chromidrosis. Hyperidrosis. Miliaria. Sudamina.

(2.) Of the sebaceous glands: Comedo. Cysts. Milium. Molluscum sebaceum. Seborrhœa.

CLASS II.

Inflammations.—Erythema. Intertrigo. Dermatitis contusiformis. Erysipelas. Pityriasis. Urticaria. Acne. Sycosis. Eczema. Dysidrosis. Pernio. Strophulus. Prairie itch. Herpes. Zoster. Hydroa. Pemphigus. Impetigo contagiosa. Ecthyma. Lichen planus. Prurigo. Lichen simplex. Psoriasis. Dermatitis exfoliativa. Anthrax. Furunculus. Hydroadenitis.

CLASS III.

Hæmorrhages.—(1.) Of connective tissue: Purpura.

CLASS IV.

Hypertrophies.—(1.) Of pigment: Chloasma. Lentigo.

(2.) Of epidermal and papillary layers: Callositas. Cornu cutaneum. Clavus. Ichthyosis. Verruca. Onychia. Paronychia. Hirsuties.

(3.) Of connective tissue: Elephantiasis. Frambœsia. Rosacea. Scleriasis. Scleroderma.

(4.) Of nail: Onychogryphosis.

(5.) Of cutis: Dermatolysis.

CLASS V.

Atrophies.—(1.) Of pigment: Leucoderma.

(2.) Of connective tissue: Morphœa.

(3.) Of hair: Alopecia.

(4.) Of nail: Atrophy of the nail.

(5.) Of cutis: Linear atrophy.

CLASS VI.

New Growths.—(1.) Of connective tissue: Fibroma. Keloid. Xanthoma. Neuroma.

(2.) Of vessels: Nævus. Telangiectasis. Lymphangioma.

(3.) Of granulation tissue: Epithelioma. Leprosy. Lupus erythematosus. Lupus vulgaris. Rhino-scleroma. Sarcoma cutis. Scrofuloderma. Syphilides.

CLASS VII.

Neuroses.—Anæsthesia. Dermatalgia. Hyperæsthesia.

CLASS VIII.

Parasitic Diseases.—(1.) Vegetable or dermatophytic: Tinea favosa. Tinea tricophytina. Tinea versicolor. Alopecia areata. Onycho-mycosis.

(2.) Animal or dermatozoic: Elephantiasis. Guinea worm disease. Mite disease. Phthiriasis. Scabies.

PART II.

THE DESCRIPTION AND TREATMENT OF SKIN DISEASES.

ACNE.

Definition.—Acne is an inflammatory disease of the sebaceous glands, caused by the retention of sebum, and characterized by the formation of papules, pustules and tubercles, which on disappearing may leave cicatrices.

Synonyms.—Varus. Ionthus. Stone-pock.

Symptomatology.—Acne, from the Greek *acme, a point*, is, next to eczema, the commonest disease of the skin. It may show itself on any part of the body, except the palms of the hands and soles of the feet, but generally selects as seats, the face and back. It affects both sexes, and is most common, between the ages of fifteen and forty-five. It occurs mostly in light complexioned young people, at the age of puberty. It is more common at this period of life, because the hair follicles and sebaceous glands are in a state of physiological hyper-activity, and hence more liable to suffer functional derangement, and to take on diseased states. It may appear either as a separate and independent affection, or exist as a complication of other follicular diseases.

The eruption usually manifests itself, in the form of pin-head or pea-sized elevations, situated around the glandular orifices, attended by more or less peri-follicular and peri-glandular inflammation. The elevations may be either light-red, dull crimson, or violaceous in color, and are usually slightly painful and tender.

The course of the disease, though at times *acute*, is usually *chronic*. When acute, it may run its course in a few days or weeks, but when chronic it may last for years. Occurring for the most part in early life, it frequently disappears spontaneously as maturity is attained.

Varieties.—The two principle varieties of acne are ACNE VULGARIS, and ACNE INDURATA. The former variety is most frequently observed in early life, and consists of pin-head or split-pea sized, discrete papules, in various degrees of development. The papules and pustules, are seldom surrounded by marked infiltration but are generally interspersed with black points (comedones). The eruption is usually confined to the face and shoulders.

The latter variety of acne, acne indurata, may follow acne vulgaris. It occurs oftenest about the twenty-fifth year, and is frequently generalized over the forehead, cheeks, *chin* and back of the neck. It consists of split-pea or small chestnut sized papules, tubercles and pustules, situated on reddened, infiltrated and hardened bases, frequently presenting the appearance of conical elevations, and often attended with pain.

The eruption is usually very chronic, often very indolent, and is apt to be attended with much disfigurement and scarring.

In debilitated states of the system, such as attains in anæmia, chlorosis, marasmus, scrofulosis, and tuberculosis, a form of the disease, termed CACHECTIC ACNE, is frequently observed. The eruption appears mostly on the trunk and extremities, and consists of indolent pin-head or bean sized, livid or violaceous, usually soft papulo-pustules, which on disappearing, leave minute cicatrices.

An acneiform eruption, to which the name, ARTIFICIAL ACNE has been applied, is occasionally produced by the constant or over-use of such substances as tar and the salts of bromine and iodine. It usually consists of reddish-brown, pin head or pea-sized papules, and differs from true acne, in that it is frequently attended by more or less inflammation of the whole skin, and by the development of pustular and furuncular lesions.

Etiology.—The causes of acne though often obscure, are frequently found in a lowered vitality, commonly associated with functional or organic derangement of the digestive and sexual systems.

ACNE VULGARIS, which is pre-eminently a disease of youth, is frequently attended with either perverted sexual habits, or a poorly regulated sexual hygiene. Menstrual irregularities, and uterine disease frequently play a not unimportant part. While various topical irritants, such as cosmetics, irritating soaps, frizzes, dyed veils, etc., in persons having irritable skin, often produce acne.

ACNE INDURATA is oftenest met with during and after adult life. In males it is frequently induced by gastric and hepatic derangements, or may be due to excessive indulgence in alcoholic liquors. In females it may be caused by gastric trouble, or by ovarian or uterine disease.

Morbid anatomy.—In acne vulgaris there is first a retention of the secretion of the sebaceous gland, and the formation of a sebaceous plug, which by blocking up the excretory duct, acts as a foreign body, and excites inflammatory hyperæmia and exudation in and around the hair follicles and glands. If the plug is not removed, pus formation, associated with painful inflammatory induration of the connective tissue about the gland, takes place. In this way the hard tubercles of acne indurata are formed. If the peri-glandular and peri-follicular inflammation is active, both the gland and the follicle may be destroyed, leaving ultimately a visible cicatrix.

Diagnosis.—The differential diagnosis of acne is exceedingly simple, if the chief characteristics and history of the disease are borne in mind. The only affections with which it is liable to be confounded are, a papulo-pustular or tubercular syphilide, rosacea, and eczema in the papular stage. From the papulo-pustular syphilide it must be distinguished by its history, by the absence of groupings of eruption and the characteristic crusts, as well as of other signs of general syphilis. From rosacea it may be distinguished by the age of the patient, by absence of itching and burning sensations, and by the color of the pimples, which are pale red or livid in acne, but brighter, and scattered over a more or less reddened patch in rosacea. In the papular stage of eczema, there is more or less interpapillary infiltration, and a disposition to scaly formation.

Treatment.—The treatment is both local and constitutional.

The diet should be light and unstimulating. Buckwheat cakes, hot-bread, nuts, cheese, fried substances, exhilarating drinks, and all sweet and rich articles of food should be avoided. In dyspeptic patients, a cup of hot water taken a half hour before meals, will often prove beneficial.

The external treatment will vary, according to the extent, obstinacy, and stage in which the disease exists.

The plugs of sebum should be removed as early as possible.

For this purpose a watch-key or what is perhaps preferable, a comedo extractor (Fig. 6) may be used. In

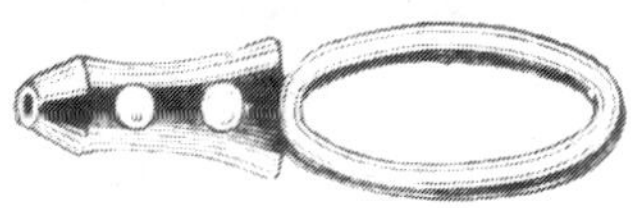

FIG. 6. COMEDO EXTRACTOR.

all inflammatory conditions the greatest benefit is obtained from five-minute applications of very hot water, two or three times per day. When the pustules are large and full, the inflammation and congestion is best relieved by passing the point of an acne lance (Fig. 7) into them, and evacuating their contents, and afterwards resorting to the hot water fomentations.

In the milder forms, and in all cases after the inflammation and congestion have somewhat subsided, the best results will generally be obtained from either a rumex lotion (rumex crispus tinct. two drachms (8),

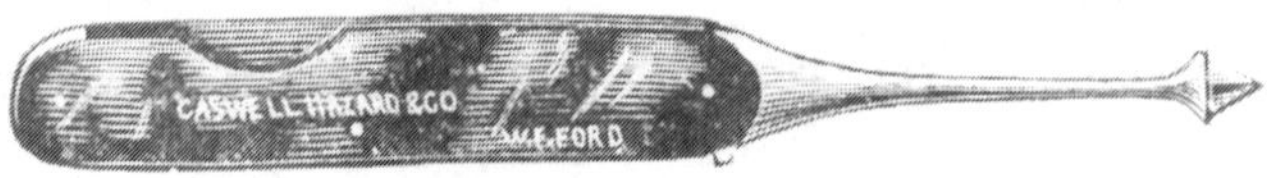

FIG. 7. ACNE LANCE.

alcohol and water, each one ounce (32), or a sulphur wash (sulphur precip. one drachm (32), glycerine, one ounce (32), aq. ros. six ounces (192).

Finely powdered sulphur, intimately mixed with three or four times its weight of rice flour or of any simple toilet powder, may be freely dusted over the face. In mild forms of acne vulgaris, this prepared sulphur powder may be used in preference to the lotions.

In acne indurata, the inflammation and induration are best relieved by freely incising the papules and pustules with the acne lance (Fig. 7), and applying hot fomentations. After the inflammation has somewhat subsided, the sulphur lotion referred to above should be employed. In obstinate cases apply nightly; an unguent made of three drachms (12.) of a five per cent oleate of mercury, and one ounce (32.) of olive oil.

The affected parts should be rubbed with a soft nail-brush and warm soap and water, every night before applying the lotions.

In indolent papular acne, associated with comedones the dermal curette (Fig. 9) may be used.

Applications of the faradic current every two or three days, and sea salt or sea water (Briggs), baths about twice a week, have occasionally rendered excellent service.

The soaps that have been found most useful, are notably, sulphur and iodide of sulphur soaps, and the Juniper tar soap.

Of internal remedies one of the following may be selected according to the indications:

Antimonium crudum.—Small, red pimples about the face, and on the right shoulder, stinging when touched. Acne in drunkards, with gastric derangements, severe thirst, and white coated tongue.

Antimonium tart.—In obstinate cases with longing for acids, and when there is a decided tendency to pustulation. The pustules are thickest on the neck and shoulders, and after discharging leave bluish-red cicatrices. May be used internally and locally.

Arsenicum.—In chronic cases when the skin is dry, rough, and dirty looking, and when the eruption is most marked on the face and extremities. Cachectic acne.

Asimina.—Itching red pimples, appearing first on the left, then on the right side. Pustular acne, with itching in the evening when undressing.

Aurum.—Red pimples on the face. Disposition to melancholy. In onanists and syphilitics. After overdosing with potassium iodide.

Baryta carb.—In obstinate cases, especially when the papules or pustules are interspersed with comedones. Adapted to scrofulous persons and to wine drinkers.

Berberis vulg.—Red, burning, gnawing pimples, sensitive to pressure, surrounded by red areolæ, and leaving brown stains. Adapted to indurated acne, associated with urinary or hæmorrhoidal troubles. In women with scanty or suppressed menstruation.

BELLADONNA.—Large, bright, red pimples on the *face*, back, and scapulæ, especially in young, full-blooded people. Fine stinging in the tips of the pimples. Worse during menstruation and pregnancy.

Bovista.—Large, scattered pimples on the forehead. Hard, red pimples, large as peas, on the chest, worse from scratching. In delicate women, with thick acrid or corrosive, greenish-yellow leucorrhœa, after the menses.

Bromine.—Indurated acne in scrofulous individuals. Aggravated by smoking. Swelling and induration of the glands of the neck.

Calcium sulphide.—Painless pimples on the nape of the neck, forehead and chin. Crusty pimples on the face in young people. Swelling and suppuration of glands.

Calcarea carb.—Acne on the face and neck, worse before menstruation. After sexual excesses. Especially in scrofulous persons.

Carbo veg.—Pimples on the nape of the neck. Red pimples on the face and chin in young persons.

Aggravated by eating butter or pork. Cachectic acne.

Causticum.—Eruption on the face, more felt than seen. Yellow color of the face. Papulous eruption between the eyebrows above the nose. Adapted to dark-haired persons.

Chelidonium maj.—Pimples and pustules in groups of three or four on the face, except the chin. Chiefly on the left side. Acne dependent upon liver derangement.

Cimicifuga.—Acne in women, dependent upon gastric ovarian or uterine derangement.

Conium mac.—In obstinate, indurated acne occurring on the face. After the suppression of the menses. Adapted to scrofulous persons, and old maids.

Eugenia jamb.—Pimples on the face which are painful for some distance around. At times useful in the indurated form.

Granatum.—Pimples on the forehead and left temple with sore pain. They suppurate and on drying leave nodules. Itching in different parts of the body as if pimples would break out.

Graphites—Acne in persons inclined to obesity; particularly females with disposition to delayed menstruation. The skin is very dry, inclined to crack, and easily tends to ulceration.

Iodine.—Indurated acne in scrofulous subjects. Adapted to young persons with dark hair and eyes, and rough, dry skin.

Kali. bich.—Face covered with a profuse eruption resembling acne. When pustules form they resemble small-pox pustules. Especially suitable for fat, light-haired persons.

KALI. CARB.—Small pimples on the face, chest, and back, with redness and swelling deficient perspiration. Aggravated during suppressed menstruation. In persons inclined to pulmonary troubles.

Kreasote.—Acne worse after menstruation, or from getting heated. Dry pimples on the forehead. Greasy pimples on the right cheek and chin.

LEDUM.—Red pimply eruption on the face. Small pimples on the root of the nose. In rheumatic persons and brandy drinkers.

Lycopodium.—Red pimples in *clusters*, between the scapulæ and on the nape of the neck. In dyspeptic individuals, inclined to constipation.

Mercurius sol.—Indolent bluish-red papules, especially on the lower extremities. Dirty yellow color of the skin, with glandular swellings. In syphilitic and scrofulous persons.

Mezereum.—Single pimples on the thighs. Red pustules with inflamed areolæ on the outer side of the extremities. In scrofulous individuals, and in persons who have already taken mercury.

Nabulus serp.—Pimples on the face, about the nose, upper lip and chin.

Natrum mur.—Acne accompanied by seborrhœa, when associated with scorbutic affections or chlorosis.

Nitric acid.—Many small pimples on the forehead, just below the hair. Painful pimples on the chin with hard, red areolæ. Skin dry and scaly. Brown-red spots on the skin. After the abuse of mercury.

NUX JUGLANS.—Variously sized reddish pimples and pustules on the face, chiefly around the mouth. Large painful blood-boils on the shoulders, and in the hepatic region. Adapted to all stages of acne.

Nux vom.—Acne with dyspepsia and constipation. After over-use of coffee, liquors or tobacco. In persons of sedentary habits.

PHOSPHORIC ACID.—Smooth, red pimples with red areolæ on the fore arm, knees and leg. Large, red pimples on the face and scapulæ, only sensitive to the touch. Acne in weakly persons, onanists, and victims of spermatorrhœa.

POTASSIUM BROMIDE.—Acne on the face, neck and shoulders, with peculiar yellow points which neither coalesce nor burst. Frontal headache at night. Adapted to both the simple and indurated forms.

POTASSIUM IODIDE.—Papulous eruption all over, but especially on the face and the shoulders. Painful sensitiveness, worse at night. In mercurial and syphilitic affections.

Pulsatilla.—Acne in pale, slender individuals. Gastric and bilious disorders. Amenorrhœa. Chlorosis. Aggravated by pastry and fat food.

Rhus tox.—Acne in drunkards, rheumatic individuals, and in persons addicted to sexual excesses.

ROBINIA.—Hard pimples which take a great while to suppurate. Great tendency of tumors to become indurated. In dyspeptics with sour stomach, worse at night. Nocturnal emissions.

Rumex crisp.—Dense rash of small red pimples.

Eruptions aggravated by wearing flannel. Itching on various parts, worse while undressing.

Sabina.—Papular eruptions during pregnancy.

Sarsaparilla.—Acne on the nose and face, worse during the menstrual period. Burning itching eruption.

Sepia—Acne on the *chin*, during pregnancy and nursing. Pimples on the mons veneris, legs and flexures of the joints. Ailments following vaccination and self-abuse.

Silicea.—Cachectic acne. Obstinate cases in scrofulous persons. Aggravated by wine drinking.

SULPHUR.—In acne vulgaris with black pores in the face. Red, itching pimples on the nose, lip, around the chin, and on the forearms. Furunculosis. Chronic cases.

Sumbul.—Smooth, small, reddish spots on the forehead. Black pores on the face.

Thuja.—Acne on the alæ nasi, worse during menstruation, and after excesses of all kinds.

Veratrum alb.—Pimples on the right labium just before menstruation.

ALOPECIA.

Alopecia or *simple baldness*, is an absence of hair, either partial or general. It is a symptom rather than a disease, and may exist as an accompaniment of a variety of affections.

ALOPECIA AREATA.

Definition.—It is a parasitic disease, characterized by the more or less sudden appearance of variously sized white, bald patches.

Synonyms.—Porrigo decalvans. Tinea decalvans.

Symptomatology.—It starts usually on the scalp, and generally from the parietal protuberances, but occasionally it commences in the beard. At times the whole body becomes affected. The disease is frequently unilateral, occurs mostly in young people, and is usually announced by the appearance of one or more nickel-sized, roundish or oval areas, devoid of hair. These are apt to extend quite rapidly, and in a few days may have attained the size of an inch or more. Other spots soon appear elsewhere, and in a short time the greater part of the side of the head may be bald. The hairs generally come out by the roots leaving a perfectly smooth polished surface, and do not break off as in *tinea tricophytina.*

At times little fine lanugo or downy hairs appear on the affected part; these, however, are seldom more than transients, and soon fall off and disappear. After this manner the disease may run indefinitely.

Etiology.—It was for some time a mooted question with dermatologists as to whether this was a parasitic affection, or merely a tropho-neurosis.

Malassez in the *Archives de Physiologie* for 1874, demonstrated its parasitic nature. He found a number of spherical and ovoid, double contoured, highly refractive bodies, among the epidermal scales. The spores were either annular or formed incomplete rings, and were seldom found on the hairs.

Treatment.—The treatment is mostly parasiticidal, and consists in epilating with a broad-lipped forceps

(Fig. 12) the marginal hairs, and applying acetic acid, tincture of cantharides, tincture of iodine, or equal parts of glycerine and tincture of capsicum, to the patch. This treatment is to be followed by an ointment of the mercuric bichloride, half to one grain (.03 to .06) to the ounce (32), applied for a fortnight, and changed morning and evening. A weak phosphorus lotion may at times render excellent service, in promoting the new growth of hair.

The principal internal remedy is *Phosphorus*, and the next *Natrum mur.* Others may be indicated for alopecia in general as follows:

Aloes.—When the hair comes out in lumps, leaving bald patches.

Arsenicum.—When it falls out in circular patches.

Calcarea carb.—When the bald spots are on the *temples.*

Calcium sulphide.—Bald spots on the head, after headaches.

Carbo veg.—Falling off of hair after severe illness, or after parturition.

Fluoric acid.—When there is a syphilitic taint.

Graphites.—Bald spots on the sides of the head.

Helleborus.—Falling off of hair from eyebrows and pudendum.

Kali carb.—Dry hair rapidly falling off with much dandruff.

Mancinella.—Falling off of the hair after severe acute diseases.

Phosphorus.—Falling out in tufts.

Phosphoric acid.—Alopecia as a result of debility.

Vinca minor.—The hair falls out in single spots, and white hair grows there.

ANÆSTHESIA.

Anæsthesia, by which is meant partial or complete *insensibility of the skin*, is encountered in such diseases, as leprosy, syphilis, hysteria, and in various affections of the brain and spinal cord. It may result from traumatism, the local use of freezing mixtures, carbolic acid and the like, or arise from the toxic effects of opium, chloroform or lead.

ANIDROSIS.

Definition.—Anidrosis may be defined as a functional disorder of the perspiratory apparatus, characterized by insufficient sweat.

It may be congenital, or exist as an accompaniment, in psoriasis, elephantiasis or icthyosis.

Treatment.—Turkish baths will be found of service. The internal remedies occasionally indicated, are:

Æthusa.—The skin has a dry, white, leathery appearance.

Natrum carb.—The skin of the whole body becomes dry and cracked.

Phosphorus.—The skin is dry and wrinkled.

Plumbum.—Dry skin, with absolute lack of perspiration.

Potassium iodide.—The skin is dried up, and rough, like hog skin.

ANTHRAX.

Definition.—Anthrax is a phlegmonous inflammation of the skin, characterized by necrosis of the cellular tissue, with suppuration, and the discharge of the necrosed masses—called cores—with pus, through corresponding sieve-like openings.

Synonym.—Carbuncle.

Symptomatology.—It generally commences with severe burning pains in the part affected, and is accompanied by more or less fever. As the disease progresses, the painful spot becomes hard and swollen and assumes a purplish hue. It is usually circumscribed, and varies in size from a fifty-cent piece to a saucer. In a few days little openings corresponding to the number of *cores*, form on the surface, and give to the part a cribriform appearance. The whole mass, now gradually sloughs away, leaving an ulcer with everted edges, which granulates slowly, and leaves when healed, a permanent, more or less pigmented cicatrix. Anthrax seldom appears before adult life and is oftener met with in men than in women. It appears most frequently on the nape of the neck, shoulders, and the lateral aspects of the hips and thighs. It is usually single, occasionally it is multiple, and not infrequently groups appear in different parts of the body. It is more frequent in winter than in summer, and occasionally displays an epidemic tendency. It may run a mild course, or it may be so severe as to terminate fatally. Pyæmia and septicæmia are its commonest complications.

Diagnosis.—Anthrax may be mistaken for erysipelas or for a collection of boils which have become confluent. It differs from erysipelas chiefly in its circumscribed character, hardness and pain. And it may be distinguished from boils by the more extensive subcutaneous necrosis, and by the more intense pain and constitutional symptoms.

Prognosis.—As anthrax is generally a serious disease the prognosis should be guarded.

Treatment.—The diet should be abundant, nutritious and easily digested, and directed mainly to keeping up the strength of the patient. In debilitated cases, a jelly made by simmering together equal parts of finely cut mutton, beef and veal may be used. Red wine or brandy and egg, or milk and egg will sometimes prove serviceable. Ventilation is important, especially if the case is severe, and the patient is confined to his bed. Platt's chlorides, a solution of carbolic acid or of thymol, or some other disinfectant, may be sprinkled upon the bed and about the room, if the carbuncle is large and open or the gangrenous sloughs extensive.

The local treatment consists in the early application of ice and salt bags to the swelling. They invariably lessen the extent of the disease. Later, if suppuration threatens, hot flax-seed meal poultices, with some antiseptic, such as carbolic acid or thymol, to lessen the risk of septic absorption and to promote the separation of the sloughs, should be applied. If the sloughing is extensive, charcoal and yeast poultices may be used. After an opening occurs or is made by the knife, the sloughs should be picked out as fast as they loosen, and the ulcer washed once or twice a day with a weak solution of carbolic acid.

Strapping with soap plaster in the early stages has been recommended. And good results have followed the injection of a saturated solution of pure carbolic acid, through the openings into the sloughing tissue, by the aid of an hypodermatic syringe.

Of internal remedies, *Arsenicum alb.* bears the palm.

Others may be used according to the indications.

Aconite.—As an occasional remedy, when there is much inflammation with high fever.

ANTHRACINUM.—Burning pain not relieved by Arsenicum. Cerebral or typhoid symptoms. *Evidences of blood poisoning.*

Apis mel.—Continued extension of the erysipelatoid inflammation with stinging burning.

ARCTIUM LAPPA has great reputation. Used both internally and locally.

ARSENICUM ALB.—Large painful and malignant carbuncles. Great prostration. Excessive burning, as from hot coals. Better from warm applications.

Belladonna.—Bright redness, with throbbing pain. When cerebral complications arise. Erysipelatous inflammation around the carbuncle.

Carbo veg.—Dark blackish appearance of the sore, with fetid discharge.

Cinchona.—When the asthenic character of the disease is well marked. Debility from excessive suppuration.

Hyoscyamus.—When there is great restlessness, caused by excessive nervous excitement. Itching around the swelling. In nervous and hysterical individuals.

Lachesis.—Bluish purplish looking carbuncles, with evidences of blood poisoning. Nightly burning, obliging one to rise and wash parts in cold water. Cerebral symptoms.

Muriatic acid.—Carbuncles in scorbutic individuals, with ulcers on the gums. Frequent desire to urinate with profuse emission of clear urine.

Nitric acid.—When there is a predisposition to anthrax.

Phytolacca.—Tendency to carbuncles, especially on the back and behind the ears.

Rhus tox.—Great restlessness. Burning itching around the carbuncle, with vertigo. Bloody, or serous, frothy, diarrhœa. Typhoid symptoms.

Secale cor.—Carbuncles on the arms. Aggravated by warm applications. Gangrenous tendency.

SILICEA.—During the process of ulceration, to promote healthy granulation.

LINEAR ATROPHY.

Definition.—Linear atrophy of the skin, is characterized by white or claret-colored, depressed scar-like streaks or spots.

Symptoms.—The *streaks*, which are the commoner form, are usually from two to five millimeters broad, and from two to several centimeters long. The *spots* may vary in size from a pins-head to a pea or larger. They both present a smooth depressed scar-like appearance, and may be either white or claret-colored. They usually occur on the pelvis brim, the glutei, and the trochanters, and less frequently on the anterior surface of the thighs or the arms.

Linear atrophy may occur at all periods of life, runs a chronic course, and seldom affects the general health of the patient.

Under the microscope, the papillary layer is found atrophied, and the corium much thinned.

It is supposed to be due to the cessation of the trophic nerve influence in localized areas.

Treatment.—*Cocculus* may be given daily to check the formation of the claret spots. *Graphites* or *Sulphur* for the white spots, and *Sabadilla* for the streaks. Usually, however, medication is unavailing. The diet should be directed to keeping up a proper and healthy state of system. Cod liver oil as a nerve food may be thought of.

ATROPHY OF THE NAIL.

Definition.—Atrophy of the nail may be either congenital or acquired, and is characterized by a deficient growth of nail substance.

Symptoms.—The nails are usually brittle, thinner than normal, and devoid of the natural lustre and smoothness. They frequently present a worm-eaten appearance, and have a deadened leaden hue.

Atrophy of the nail may exist as a local affection, or as is more generally the case, occur as a result of other diseases, such as eczema, psoriasis, or syphilis.

Treatment.—The principal internal remedy for simple atrophy of the nail is Silicea.

BAKER'S ITCH.

Definition.—Baker's itch is an inflammation of the skin induced by the irritant action of flour. *See* eczema.

BALDNESS.

Definition.—*See* Alopecia.

BARBER'S ITCH.

Definition.—*See* Tinea Tricophytina.

BOILS.

Definition.—*See* Furuncle.

BRICK-LAYER'S ITCH.

Definition.—Bricklayer's itch, is an inflammation of the skin, excited by the irritant action of lime. *See* Eczema.

BROMIDROSIS.

Definition.—Bromidrosis is a functional disorder of the sweat glands, characterized by offensive sweat.

Synonyms.—Osmidrosis. Offensive sweating.

Symptoms.—It may be either general or local. The

former is usually associated with some constitutional disease. Local bromidrosis is commonly located in the feet, axillæ, and genital regions. The hands and feet are frequently cold, and present a bluish appearance, due to inactive circulation. Sometimes the disorder is due to the saturation of long worn socks and boots. The odor varies, being at times almost imperceptible, and in other cases so strong as to be truly disgusting.

An osmidrosis may exist, as a symptom in general diseases. Fox mentions the "rank" sweat in rheumatism, "the putrid" sweat in scurvy, the "musky" sweat in chronic peritonitis, the "mouldy" sweat in itch, the "sweet" sweat in syphilis, the "stale beer" sweat in scrofula, and the "fresh-baked brown bread" sweat in intermittent fever.

Treatment.—Local bromidrosis is often very difficult of cure. The most thorough cleanliness should be observed. The parts may be washed with plenty of soap—juniper-tar soap is the best—morning and evening, then dried and powdered with starch. Sea water baths (using Brigg's concentrated sea-water) at night prove useful in some cases.

The internal remedy may be selected from the following:

Artemisia vulg.—Odor of garlic.

Baptisia.—Fœtid sweat. Frequent sweat from small of the back in all directions.

Belladonna.—Sweat on covered parts. It stains the clothing and has an empyreumatic smell.

Bryonia.—Sour or oily sweat night and day. Sweat in short spells, and only on single parts.

Cantharis.—Sweating on the genitals. Sweat smells like urine.

Carbo veg.—Profuse, putrid or sour sweat. Foot-sweat, excoriating the toes.

Cinchona.—Profuse, sickly smelling sweats. Exhausting night-sweats.

Colocynth.—Noctural sweat on the head and extremities, smelling like urine, and causing itching of the skin.

Conium mac.—Strong, fœtid, acrid, irritating sweat. Offensive odor without perspiration.

Dulcamara.—Fœtid sweat with copious discharge of limpid urine. Offensive night and morning sweat.

Graphites.—Sour, offensive, yellow staining sweat. Profuse foot-sweat. Soreness and rawness between the toes after walking.

Ledum.—Putrid, sour sweat, at night. Itching of the body.

Lycopodium.—Sweat smelling like onions. Sweat from the least exertion.

Nitric acid.—Odor like horse's urine.

Nux vom.—Odor of musty straw, night and morning.

Petroleum.—Fœtid sweat in the axilla. Tenderness of the feet as if bathed in foul moisture. Tendency of skin to fester and ulcerate.

Phosphorus.—Sweat smelling of sulphur. Sweat mostly on the head, hands and feet.

Rheum.—Sour smelling sweats.

Rhododendron.—Spicy smelling sweat with formication and itching of the skin. Offensive smelling sweat in the axilla.

Sepia.—Sweat sour, or like elder blossoms. Offensive foot-sweat. During exercise.

SILICEA.—*Offensive foot-sweats*, with rawness between the toes.

Solanum tub.—When in bed, the sweat has the odor of potatoes.

Stannum.—Mouldy, musty, smelling sweat.

STAPHYSAGRIA.—Sweat smelling like rotten eggs. Uterine diseases.

Sulphur.—Sweat has a burnt odor.

Veratrum alb.—Bitter smelling sweat, staining the linen yellow.

CALLOSITAS.

Definition.—Callositas consists of an abnormal deposit of epidermal cells, forming a yellowish or whitish, nickel-sized, horny, elevated patch, occurring especially on parts exposed to pressure or friction.

Synonyms.—Callus. Callosity. Tylosis. Tyloma.

Symptoms.—It is observed on the hands of mechanics and laboring men. On the foot it is caused by the friction of the boot, and appears mostly on the ball of the great toe, and on the outside of the little toe. It is found more in men than in women.

Diagnosis.—It differs from clavus or corn in its diffuse character, in the absence of pain, and in its involving only the outer portions of the epidermis.

Treatment.—Occasionally it disappears spontaneously. If it proves a source of annoyance it may be removed by a knife (Fig. 8) or rasping, otherwise it is advisable not to interfere with it. When the soles become greatly hardened, and are fissured and painful relief can be obtained by wearing constantly, within the stocking, oiled silk cut a little larger than the sole.

Graphites and *Silicea* are respectively the main remedies for callosities on the hands and feet.

CANCER.

The main variety of cancer with which the dermatologist, strictly speaking, has to deal, is the *epithelial*. The others belong to the province of the surgeon. *See* Epithelioma.

CARBUNCLE.

See anthrax.

CHLOASMA.

Definition.—Chloasma is a discoloration of the skin, of internal origin, characterized by the formation of round or oval patches, nickel-sized or larger, having a yellowish or brownish color.

Synonyms.—Liver spots. Moth.

Symptoms.—It occurs more in women than in men, and is situated chiefly about the face and neck. It usually appears in the form of crescentic patches on the forehead and temples, also about the mouth. In women it is frequently found associated with and dependent upon some physiological or pathological change in the uterus. In men it sometimes occurs in connection with tuberculosis, and after long-continued malarial diseases.

Treatment.—Local applications are of temporary benefit. The one most commonly used is the mercuric bichloride lotion of the strength of two grains (.13) to the ounce (32.) of the emulsion of almonds. It may be painted on the parts night and morning. The oleate of copper ointment, prepared by dissolving one drachm (4.) of the salt of oleate of copper in sufficient oleo-palmitic acid to make a soft ointment, is also of service.

The internal remedies most useful in chloasma are:

Argentum nit.—Slight brown spots on the upper part of the chest and on the hands. Peculiar discoloration of the skin from bronze color to black.

Antimonium crud.—Brown liver-colored spots on both shoulders.

Caulophyllum.—In nervous and hysterical women, and when associated with painful menstruation.

Ferrum met.—In chlorotic individuals.

GUARANA.—Yellow spots on the temples. Liver spots on the arms.

LAUROCERASUS.—Hepatic spots on the face.

LYCOPODIUM.—Hepatic spots on the arms. Several brown spots on inner side of both thighs.

Nux vom.—Chloasma dependent upon liver derangement.

PETROLEUM.—Brown spots on the wrists. Yellow spots on the arms.

SEPIA.—Yellow streak like a saddle on the nose and cheeks. In pregnant or nervous women.

Sulphur.—Hepatic spots on the back and chest. Yellow and brown spots.

Woorari.—This remedy has been used with benefit.

CHROMIDROSIS.

Definition.—Chromidrosis is a functional disorder of the sweat glands, giving rise to a colored perspiration.

Synonym.—Colored sweating.

Symptoms.—Blue, yellow and red sweat have been observed. It occurs mostly in hypochondriacs and in nervous and hysterical females. The secretion is usually fitful in character, and may be excited by emotional conditions.

Treatment.—*Nux vom.*, is the most important remedy.

CLAVUS.

Definition.—Clavus is a small, usually split-pea sized, flat horny formation, more or less deeply seated, and painful on pressure.

Synonym.—Corn.

Symptoms.—It may be either *hard* or *soft*. A hard corn is usually located on an outer surface, and a soft corn is generally located between the toes, where the parts are kept moist. A corn resembles a callosity when hard, and a wart when soft. It is almost invariably due to wrongly fitting coverings for the feet.

Treatment.—First of all the patient must consent to

wear easily fitting shoes or boots. The corn may be gotten rid of by soaking it in warm water or poulticing it over night, after which the outer layers may be removed with the corn knife (Fig. 8) After continuing this treatment for several successive nights, the formation will be softened to such an extent, that it can be removed without pain.

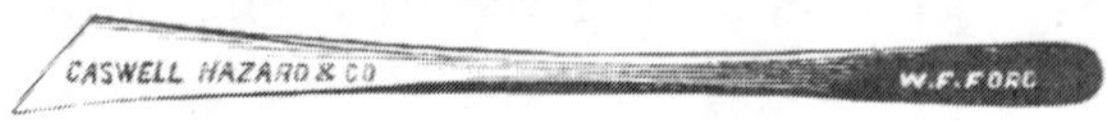

FIG. 8. CORN KNIFE.

Repeated dressing of the parts with narrow, short, nicely adjusted strips of Maw's moleskin plaster, after the corn has been thoroughly macerated and the projecting portions removed with the corn knife, are also of service.

Flexible or arnicated colloid may be used as a dressing for painful soft corns.

Ringed corn plasters often prove valuable aids in protecting the corns.

If the corns are inflamed and painful, a veratrum viride or arnica lotion, one part to ten, may be resorted to instead of the poultices.

A lotion consisting of one drachm (4.) of salicylic acid, ten grains (.66) of extract of cannabis indica, and one ounce (32.) of collodion, applied with a camel's hair brush once or twice a day has been used with great success in removing corns.

ANTIMONIUM CRUDUM, is the principal internal remedy for *hard* corns, and *Sulphur* for the *soft* variety.

COMEDO.

Definition.—Comedo is a disorder of the sebaceous glands, characterized by small black-topped sebaceous points.

Synonym.—Acne punctata.

Etiology.—Comedo depends largely upon gastro-intestinal or genital irritation.

Symptoms.—Comedones, vulgarly styled worms or grubs, are small, hardened plugs of sebaceous matter contained within the cavity and ducts of the glands. They vary in size from a pin-point to a pin-head. The disease shows itself generally on the forehead, cheeks and chin. It appears mostly in young people, between the ages of fifteen and twenty-five, and is a frequent accompaniment of acne.

In the substance of the mass of retained sebum which may be squeezed out of the gland, a living and innocent grub, first discovered by Henle in 1841, and called the acarus folliculorum, is frequently, though not always observed.

Diagnosis.—It differs from milium in that the sebaceous duct in comedo is patulous, in milium it is closed. The face looks as if sprinkled with gunpowder in comedo, in milium it appears studded with white millet-seed like points.

Prognosis.—If left to itself, comedo rarely runs longer than four or five years. Matrimony is said to hasten its departure.

Treatment.—The diet should in the majority of cases be regulated so as to exclude oily and fatty foods and pastry.

In some cases, however, cod liver oil may be needed.

The individual comedos should be squeezed out with a watch key or the comedo extractor (Fig. 6), and a sulphur lotion, composed of sublimed sulphur two drachms (8.) and alcohol one ounce (32.) applied and allowed to remain on all night.

The principal internal remedies are BARYTA CARB. and SELENIUM. Others may be indicated as follows:

Belladonna.—Comedos in young full-blooded people.

Cicuta.—Black spots on the skin.

Digitalis.—Black comedos on the skin of the face, which suppurate.

Mezereum.—Small comedos on the nose and cheeks.

Nitric acid.—Black sweat pores in the skin of the face.

Sabina.—Comedos that can be easily pressed out, in the cheeks and about the nose.

Sulphur.—Blackish pores in the face.

Sumbul.—Numerous black pores on the face. Skin pale.

CONDYLOMATA.

Definition.—Condylomata are contagious lesions peculiar to syphilis, and consist of round, oval or oblong, pale or rosy, usually elevated spots, covered with a whitish pellicle.

Synonyms.—Mucous patches. Mucous tubercles. Plaques muqueuses.

Symptomatology.—They are moist lesions, which may appear at any period of syphilis, but are more common during the early stages. They vary in size from a pin's head to a fifty cent piece or larger, and select as seats, notably the muco-cutaneous surfaces. They are seen mostly about the anus, throat, mouth and genitals, and beneath the mammæ, and usually appear upon the skin in connection with the papular syphilide. They are superficial and of a grayish-white color in the mouth, but raised and of a reddish color about the genitals. Their secretion is glairy and intensely contagious.

Treatment.—Keep the parts clean and dry. If the excrescences are troublesome, excise them with the knife and afterwards apply a mercuric bichloride lotion, strength one to two grains (.066 to 0.133) to the ounce (32.) of water.

The principal internal remedy is *Thuja*. Other remedies may be indicated as follows:

CINNABAR.—Fan-shaped fig-warts accompanied by tetter. In scrofulous infants and children.

Euphrasia.—Fig-warts at the anus.

MERCURIUS COR.—Dry fig-warts, or else fig-warts accompanied by acrid discharges. Soft, flat condylomata.

Mercurius nit.—Filiform fig-warts.

Mercurius precip. ruber.—Fissured condylomata.

Mercurius sol.—Conical fig-warts. Small, itching pimples which ulcerate and become incrusted. Mild types.

NITRIC ACID.—Pediculated and pen-shaped, moist condylomata. Fig-warts on the glans.

Sabina.—Condylomata attended with itching and burning.

Sarsaparilla.—Flat fig-warts.

Staphysagria.—Cock's comb shaped fig-warts.

Sulphur.—Soft, spongy fig-warts.

THUJA.—Cauliflower excrescences. Condylomata on the penis, vulva and about the anus. Broad, flat condylomata. After iritis, tubercles or warty excrescences on the iris.

CORNU CUTANEUM.

Definition.—A cutaneous horn is a curved, conical-ridged, usually brownish, corneous eminence, formed of dense, closely compressed columns of epithelia.

Synonyms.—Cutaneous horn. Horny excrescence.

Symptomatology.—Cutaneous horns commonly develop upon the head, but sometimes upon the penis, and other portions of the body. They are usually of small size; occasionally they measure several inches in length. Their growth is attended with little or no pain.

Treatment.—At times the horn is shed spontaneously, generally it is necessary to excise the entire structure with a portion of the skin from which it grows.

DERMATALGIA.

Definition.—Dermatalgia is an affection of the skin characterized by pain, and is unattended by structural change.

Synonym.—Cutaneous neuralgia.

Symptomatology.—It attacks principally parts that are covered with hair and occurs oftener in women than men. The affected parts are very sensitive to external impressions, and the pain may be continuous or intermittent, slight or severe. It is usually of a burning character, worse at night, and may last a week or longer.

Dermatalgia is to be differentiated from pruritus and cutaneous hyperæsthesia.

Treatment.—The galvanic current, at times affords magic relief. Local application of the rubber bag filled with very hot water is also useful.

The following remedies may be compared: Baryta, Bell., Bryonia, Cinchona, Ferrum, Manganum, Nux mosch., Nux vom., Phos. Sepia, Spigelia, Sulph., Veratrum, etc.

DERMATITIS CONTUSIFORMIS.

Definition.—Dermatitis contusiformis may be defined as an acute affection, characterized by oval or round purplish nodules, varying from the size of a hickory nut to that of a fist.

Synonym.—Erythema nodosum.

Symptomatology.—The attack is generally ushered in by slight febrile disturbance, more or less loss of appetite, malaise, and wandering rheumatic pains. The nodules are developed suddenly, and appear in crops of rarely less than a dozen in number. They are firm and hard, tender to pressure, and reddish or purplish in color as they are first formed, but grow darker and softer as they grow older. They develop mostly on the anterior surface of the leg, with their long diameter running lengthwise of the limb. Occasionally they appear on the arms and face, and are marked by a dark red periphery. They never suppurate, but disappear by absorption, and fade away in color like bruises. They are frequently accompanied by burning pain and considerable constitutional disturbance.

The disease is seen mostly in young persons, especially females, and is often associated with rheumatism and chorea.

It occurs more frequently in spring and fall, seldom lasts longer than two or three weeks, and tends to spontaneous recovery. Relapses are apt to take place.

Etiology.—Dermatitis contusiformis is supposed to be due to embolism of the cutaneous vessels, and is somewhat allied to purpura.

Treatment.—The local treatment consists in cold or warm arnica or hamamelis dressings, and if the part affected is the limb, a horizontal position should be maintained.

RHUS VENENATA, is the principal internal remedy. Others may be used according to the indications.

Apis mel.—Inflamed erysipelatous appearance of the nodules. Stinging, burning pains. Relieved by cold dressings.

ARNICA.—Yellow, blue, and reddish-blue spots. Pain as if beaten. In lying-in women.

PTELEA TRIF.—Red spots on the lower extremities, alike in position on both. After an hour or so change to purple color. The spots become dirty yellow, and leave the appearance of a bruise.

Rhus venenata.—Red spots from half an inch to two

inches in diameter, especially on the legs below the knees, painful and changing color into bluish then greenish yellow.

DERMATITIS EXFOLIATIVA.

Definition.—Dermatitis exfoliativa, may be defined as a disease usually involving the whole surface, and characterized by a highly reddened skin, and the abundant exfoliation of epidermis in the form of large thin whitish flakes.

Synonym.—Pityriasis rubra.

Symptomatology.—Dermatitis exfoliativa has been generally described under the name pityriasis rubra, an unfortunate term which is apt to mislead, as the scales are not *branny* as in ordinary *pityriasis*, but *flakey*.

It commonly begins in the form of small and red flakey patches which rapidly increase in size, unattended by either thickening of the skin or itching. The flakes vary in size, from a nickle to several centimeters in diameter, and when removed, leave the skin red and shining. Handfuls of these armor-like plates may be shed in twenty-four hours.

It is a rare disease, occurs mostly in adult males, and may be either acute or chronic. It involves the papillary layer alone, and is supposed to be due to a disturbance of the trophic nerves.

Diagnosis.—It is most likely to be confounded with eczema in the squamous stage, psoriasis, pemphigus foliaceus and lichen ruber.

Treatment.—Soothing local applications, such as bran baths or a decoction of walnut leaves followed by oily inunctions, and later by oil of white birch, are important aids.

The internal treatment should be directed if need be towards bringing about a healthy condition of the system.

ARSENICUM ALB. is the principal remedy.

Other remedies occasionally indicated are: Arsenicum iodide, Kali ars., Piper methysticum, Clematis, Graphites, Phosphorus and Sulphur iodide.

DERMATOLYSIS.

Definition—Dermatolysis consists of an hypertrophy of the connective tissue elements of the skin, assuming the form of pendulous or purse-like folds.

Synonym.—Cutis pendula.

Symptomatology.—It seldom appears before the age of puberty, though occasionally it is congenital. It runs a slow course, and may be confined to certain regions or appear on any part of the body.

Treatment.—If the folds are large they may be ligatured and excised.

Ammonium bromide has some reputation in arresting the disease. Staphysagria and Carbo animalis may be studied.

DYSIDROSIS.

Definition.—Dysidrosis may be defined as an inflammation of the sweat structures of the hands and feet, and is characterized by redness and swelling of the parts with distension of the sweat ducts in the form of sago-like points, and the development of bullæ.

Symptomatology.—It appears more in summer than in winter, and attacks symmetrically the sides and palmar surfaces of the fingers, the palms, and sometimes the soles of the feet. It selects as its victims the nervously debilitated, and tends to run a definite course of two or three weeks duration. Usually after the disease has existed for some time, the epidermis becomes macerated, and peels off, leaving the skin sore and painful.

Treatment.—The local treatment consists in using soothing applications, notably alkaline baths to which a little starch has been added, and afterward wrapping the parts up in carron oil.

Clematis and *Natrum sulph.*, are the most important internal remedies.

ECTHYMA.

Definition.—Ecthyma is characterized by the development of large, isolated painful pustules, situated upon hard and inflamed bases, and followed by dark-brown crusts, which on falling leave temporary scars.

Symptomatology.—The pustules are roundish or oval, flattened, of a yellow or yellowish-red color, and are surrounded by a bright red areola. Slight febrile disturbance usually precedes their outbreak. After a few days the contents of the pustules dry to form flat dark brown crusts, which when removed leave extensive excoriations, and resultant temporary scars and pigmentation. Ecthyma may occur at any time of life and selects as its victims the badly nourished and cachectic. Scratching often plays an important part in its causation and continuance. The neck, shoulders and extremities are its most frequent seats.

It is a superficial lesion, and rarely extends beyond the papillary layer.

Diagnosis.—It may be confounded with eczema and impetigo contagiosa, but is more apt to be mistaken for the large, flat, *pustular syphilide.* Ecthyma, however, develops mcre rapidly, has more heat and pain, and has slight ulceration and brownish crusts; while the syphilide has a more or less deep ulcer, with abrupt edges, and a blackish crust.

Prognosis.—Ecthyma is always curable and displays no disposition to relapse.

Treatment.—The patient should be well hygiened and given a good generous diet. The crusts may be removed after soakings with oil, and the affected parts dressed with a weak white precipitate ointment—five (.33) to ten (.66) grains to the ounce (32.) of cosmoline. After the pustules burst, if the ulcers show but little tendency to heal, a weak carbolized wash may be used.

The appropriate internal remedy may be selected from the following:

Antimonium crud.—Pustules on the face in fat people. Yellowish or brownish scabs on the face. Desire for acids.

Arsenicum alb.—Red or white pustules with intense burning. Painful, black pustules. Thick crusts leaving well marked scars in cachectic individuals.

Belladonna.—Pustules surrounded by a whitish areola. Burning and itching with great sensibility to touch.

Cicuta.—Confluent pustules about the face, forming yellow crusts.

Cyclamen.—Pustules on the feet and toes.

Croton tig.—Confluent pustules with oozing and burning. Greyish brown crusts on the abdomen.

Kali bich.—Pustules all over the body having a small brown scab on top. Pustules at the root of the nails, spreading over the hands. Pustules resembling small-pox. In light-haired people.

Kreasote.—Large pustules with violent itching towards evening. Ulcers on the face and chin.

Mercurius.—Suppurating pustules, which either run together discharging an acrid fluid, or which remain sore, become hollow, and afterwards raised and cicatrized. Ulcers bleed easily.

Nitric acid.—Feeling as of a splinter sticking into the pustules when touching them.

Petroleum.—Itching and burning pustules. Great lassitude.

Piper nigrum.—Large pustules leaving marks on the face.

Rhus tox.—Pustules seated upon a red base, with much itching and burning. Worse at night and in cold and stormy weather.

Secale.—Pustules on the arms and legs, with tendency to gangrene. In cachectic, scrawny females with rough skin.

Silicea.—Ecthymatous pustules all over the body, sensitive to contact. Pustules on the back part of the head. Burning and soreness after scratching.

Sulphur.—Dry, thick yellow scabs over the whole body. Itching pustules on the scalp, painful to the touch.

TARTAR EMET.—Large, round, full burning pustules with red areolæ, forming in two days, and leaving deep scars.

Thuja.—Suppurating pustules upon the lower extremities.

Cistus and Nux juglans may at times be indicated.

ECZEMA.

Definition.—Eczema may be defined as an acute or chronic simple inflammation of the skin, characterized by an erythematous, papular, vesicular or pustular eruption which gives rise to a moist reddened surface discharging a gummy serous fluid that stiffens as it dries, accompanied with burning and itching.

Synonyms.—Salt rheum. Moist tetter. Milk crust.

Symptomatology.—Eczema may be either acute or chronic. It may commence abruptly or gradually, and may run its course in a few weeks or last for months or years.

The *acute form* is frequently though not always ushered in by more or less febrile disturbance, lassitude and loss of appetite, which are soon followed by an eruption of one or more reddish patches of variable size, accompanied by heat and burning. In a day or two or at times even in a few hours, little pin points are seen on the reddened surface, and vesicles make their appearance, attended with more or less itching. The vesicles are small and closely aggregated. They are made up mostly of serum, containing a few leucocytes and a little fibrin, and rarely last longer than twenty-four or forty-eight hours. The *itching* is now the most prominent subjective symptom. The period of redness and vesiculation is called the FIRST STAGE.

As the vesicles mature, the clear serum becomes cloudy, and pustules are formed which either rupture spontaneously or from friction. Usually in proportion to the amount of leucocytes contained in the effusion, the disease will be either decidedly vesicular or decidedly pustular. After rupture the contents of the pustules dry upon the surface in the form of characteristic *yellowish-green scabs.* On removal of the scabs or crusts a moist reddened surface becomes visible. This is the SECOND or EXUDATIVE stage, and may be of indefinite duration. The advancing border of the disease may be marked, either by the formation of new papules and vesicles, or by the simple exfoliation of the stratum corneum. This latter phenomenon may be explained by the fact, that succeeding the primary congestion, there is an exudation from the vessels, which may instead of lifting up the layers to form vesicles, ooze through, and float the corneal layer of cells.

After a time the exudation lessens, the crusts grow thinner, the effusion ceases, the surface becomes dry, white scales take the place of crusts, and the disease is in the THIRD STAGE.

Occasionally the skin becomes much infiltrated and thickened, or in more aggravated forms takes on a decided tendency to fissure. If, however, the patches tend to recovery, the scales become finer and more adherent, and the skin gradually returns to its natural condition without a scar.

According as the disease is mild or severe, or accompanied by an amount of pustulation and crusting out of proportion to the extent of the inflammation present, it has received the names of *E. simplex*, *E. rubrum* and *E. impetiginosum.*

Not infrequently the disease instead of going through its typical course stops short at, or aborts during any one of the stages of development. Thus the eruption may remain erythematous from first to last (*E. erythematosum*). Or the disease may pass rapidly through the condition of hyperæmia to the development of small red papules, and then linger (*E. papulosum.*) Or again the papules may quickly become vesicles (*E. vesiculosum*); or the inflammation may pass to a pustular form (*E. pustulosum.*) Or lastly, the disease may run through all its stages or pass over any one of them, and remain stationary indefinitely in the third stage, (*E. squamosum.*)

ACUTE ECZEMAS may vary somewhat in their general characters, according to their location and the temperament of the patient.

In nervo-bilious subjects they tend to become irritable, in gouty subjects they are apt to be inflammatory, and in scrofulous individuals they run speedily and freely to the formation of pus.

When occurring on the *scalp*—a common seat in infants—the disease passes rapidly through the erythematous and vesicular to the pustular stage, and is followed by the formation of thick greenish-yellow crusts, covering a raw red and cracked surface. The sero-purulent discharge glues the hairs together and a dense matted crust may be produced. This form may persist for years if neglected, and is seldom attended by much itching. Subcutaneous abscesses and glandular enlargements are not infrequently met with in strumous children.

On the *face* the eruption is often symmetrical and may be present in different stages. In adults it tends to linger in the erythematous stage, and usually proves a very stubborn form of the disease. In children, eczema in this locality has been given the title of *crusta lactea.*

On the eyelids it is frequently very troublesome, and is often confounded with inflammation of the Meibomian glands. The margins of the lids are thickened and red, and there may be partial or complete loss of the eyelashes.

On the nostrils it generally terminates in the formation of a thick scab.

On the lips it may be red, scaly or moist, and is often attended by marked œdema with fissures. Erythematous eczema about the mouth is apt to prove stubborn, and tends to become chronic.

On the *ears* there is generally considerable inflammation and swelling. The vesicles may be well developed, but proceed to early pustulation. The discharge either drips away constantly or dries and forms stalactiform crusts. Small abscesses may at times develop.

In the *axillæ*, enlargement of the axillary glands with the formation of abscesses is frequently observed.

On the *nipples* it is usually accompanied by severe pruritus and a copious discharge of yellowish or reddish serum.

On the *genitals* there is commonly considerable attendant heat and redness. Moisture is always a prominent symptom. In females it affects chiefly the labia majora and usually takes the severe form (*E. rubrum*). Appearing about the anus it leads to the formation of painful itching fissures.

On the *arms*, *legs* and *thighs* it proves one of the most obstinate forms. It is attended by intolerable itching, and is apt to pass through the erythematous and be prolonged in the pustular stage.

The *flexures of the joints* and the *clefts of the nates* are oftener affected with the severer type (*E. rubrum*) than other parts of the body.

On the *hands* and *feet* it is usually symmetrical, and frequently assumes the fissured form with but little exudation and crusting. Local irritants are the most common causes of eczema restricted to the hands and feet.

On the *umbilicus* it assumes either the severe (*E. rubrum*) or pustular (*E. impetiginosum*) form or is marked by considerable œdema.

In young children "scratch marks" are scattered with more or less profusion over the affected surface.

CHRONIC ECZEMAS may either start as primary affections, or with acute or sub-acute symptoms, the disease halting either in the second, or more frequently in the third stage. They are more common than the acute variety, and may be said to exist whenever eczemas take on definite lines of action or show a tendency to repeat themselves, and are accompanied by secondary changes. They usually involve a limited surface of the skin; exceptionally they invade the entire surface of the body. They are prone to recurrent exacerbations of an acute grade, and are generally attended by more or less itching.

On the *scalp* chronic eczema is frequently accompanied by falling off of the hair. Adults of a lymphatic and scrofulous habit, and especially women at the meno-pause, are apt to be troubled with this lingering form. It tends to spread to the ears and eyebrows, and may be followed by warty thickening of the skin. Squamous or scaly eczema is apt to be attended by itching and the constant shedding of scales.

On the *cheeks*, *chin* and *upper lip* it is very intractable. The parts are more infiltrated than in the acute form and may be covered with bran-like scales. Erythematous eczema about the mouth is very rebellious.

On the *ears* it is very obstinate when it attacks females at the climacteric. Chronic eczema of the auditory canal is not infrequent. The parts are usually moist, thickened and itchy. Not infrequently they are fissured, especially at the reflection of the auricle from the mastoid process.

On the *nasal mucous membrane* it may form crusts which adhere for years and give rise to annual returns of erysipelas of the face.

On the *mammæ* it may result in the formation of fissures and abscesses. Glycosuria is a common accompaniment.

On the *perineum* and *anus* there is always more or less moisture with a decided tendency to fissure.

On the *genitals* thickening of the scrotum is apt to take place. Occasionally the penis is affected. Not infrequently there is severe itching.

On the *hands* and *feet* it sometimes commences by the appearance of fissures which are red and painful, and give forth a viscid secretion which dries into scales.

On the *legs*, especially in old people, it is prone to take on an inflammatory state, with a tendency to the formation of ulcers. Infiltration is always a common feature of chronic eczema. Chronic hard patches often occur about the ankles and prove very rebellious.

Etiology.—Eczema, attacks more frequently light, florid complexioned individuals, and is a commoner affection in this country, than in Europe. In Chicago, according to my experience, it constitutes about forty-five per cent of the entire number of skin diseases.

Like the individual who makes a failure in life, eezema usually travels, from head to foot as age advances. It appears more particularly on the head in infancy and youth, descends to the trunk and genitals as adult life approaches, and appears on the lower limbs as its victim is tottering to the grave.

Some individuals are so constituted that their skins are ever ready, on the slightest provocation to take on diseased states. In such persons anything which tends to lower the average degree of health, is apt, other things being equal, to give rise to an attack of eczema.

Dyspepsia in its influence through mal-assimilation, is after this manner, a very potent cause. Diseased states of the kidneys or bowels, and an inactive skin, whereby the proper excretory functions are interfered with, frequently produce and keep up the disease. Gouty and rheumatic patients are prone to attacks of eczema. In children, dentition plays an important part. Pregnancy at times occasions an outbreak. Blacksmiths, grocers, bakers, washerwomen, and workers in lime, from the irritating nature of their employment, are liable to the types known as grocer's, bakers's washerwoman's, etc., itch.

At times eczema becomes substitutive. And so occasionally it may be seen to disappear from the skin in connection with the development of a bronchitis, leucorrhœa, or intestinal catarrh or vice versa. Its disappearance is thus looked upon as a consequence, not a cause of the latter.

Of local causes or those which give rise to *artificial*

eczema may be mentioned; excessive use of mercury, croton tig., cantharides, mustard, rhus ven. and rhus tox. strong potash soaps, and the contact of aniline dyes and pediculi. An attack may sometimes occur from the injudicious use of Turkish and Russian baths.

Eczema is due to faulty innervation, by which cell proliferation and capillary congestion, with their consequences are produced. The papillary layer is its principal seat and the *modus operandi* of its development is as follows: An exudation of serum takes place from the congested vessels, which floats the over-supply of new cells, and the two push on to the rete from the papillary layer, separate the cell elements of the stratum malpighii and stratum lucidum, and uplift the cuticle so as to form first papules, and then vesicles.

Diagnosis.—The diagnosis of typical eczema presents but little difficulty. It is only in the irregular and imperfectly developed cases that mistakes may arise.

In the erythematous stage it may be confounded with erythema, but the subsequent course of the disease soon disperses any doubt. In the papular stage, it at times resembles lichen. Lichen affects particularly the outside of the limbs, and is a decidedly *plastic* inflammation, while eczema is a *serous* one. In the vesicular stage, eczema, herpes, zoster, and scabies, may bear considerable resemblance. The points of difference are: the vesicles of herpes are larger than those of eczema, and appear mostly on the face and genitals. The eczematous vesicles may be irregularly distributed over the body. Eczema is never attended by the neuralgic pain of zoster, and the eruption does not follow the course of the nerves. It is seldem accompanied by the intense *nightly* itching, so characteristic of scabies. The presence of acari, and the rapid disappearance of the disease under parasiticidal treatment, will at once decide the question. In the stage of incrustation, it may be mistaken for impetigo contagiosa and tinea favosa. The crusts of impetigo contagiosa, are superficial and appear as if stuck on. Those of favus are cup-shaped and of a sulphur-yellow color. Eczema crusts are greenish-yellow.

In the squamous stage, it may be confounded with psoriasis, seborrhœa, dermatitis exfoliativa, and the foliaceous variety of pemphigus. Psoriasis never has a history of discharge, and the scales are silvery white. In seborrhœa, the scales are oily and larger than in eczema. Dermatitis exfoliativa presents large, thin easily detached "flakes," which when removed leave a dry, reddish, glazed surface. Foliaceous pemphigus starts from bullæ, and the scales are thick and parchment-like. Eczema of the breast differs from "Paget's Disease" in that the latter is an epithelial degeneration which frequently ends in cancer.

The diagnosis of the principal diseases of the scalp is given in the following table arranged by Morris:

ECZEMA.	SEBORRHŒA.	PSORIASIS.	VESICO-PUSTULAR SYPHILIDE.	TINEA TONSURANS.	FAVUS.
1. Most frequent in children, in the debilitated or strumous.	1. Usually in adults.	1. Most often in healthy persons, rarely in strumous.	1. Usually in adults only.	1. Frequent in children.	1. No special proneness in strumous.
2. Often attacks the whole scalp. Ulcers, if any, superficial; crusts thick, yellowish, brittle; pus, epithelium and granular matter. Seated on red, infiltrated, moist, often, excoriated surface, which shades off gradually into healthy skin and itches excessively.	2. Crusts are thin, oily, can be kneaded into masses; consist chiefly, of sebum and epithelium on a smooth, oily surface; not, or only slightly, red, and non-excoriated or infiltrated; itching only slight.	2. Eruption usually white, scaly, and silvery; dry from onset and throughout course; red base, only slightly infiltrated, and itching only slight.	2. In small patches usually; often deep ulcers with sloughy bases.	2. Patches usually circular, deficient in hair; crusts, etc., not necessarily present; itching slight.	2. Round, dry, sulphur yellow, cup-shaped crusts, penetrated by dull brittle hairs, with abrupt edges and often bald patches.
3. Syphilitic history and phenomena only accidental, if present at all.	3. Usually no specific phenomena.	3. Usually no specific history.	3. Usually a history of primary syphilis, and presence of alopecia, nocturnal pains, etc.		
4. Distinct eczema often on other parts of body, on flexor surfaces or behind the ears.	4. Usually only slight, oily crusting on face near scalp.	4. Well-marked scaly patches, usually present on extensor surfaces of elbows and knees.	4. Syphilides, squamous, pustular, tubercular, etc., with coppery color, usually present on body.	4. Ringworm of body (tinea circinata) often present.	4. Cupped yellow crusts may be found on hairy parts of the body.
5. Hair healthy, occasionally falling out; no parasite.	5. Hairs often drop out.	5. Hairs only slightly affected.	5. Hairs fall out freely, and incurable alopecia may result.	5. Hairs twisted, thickened, whitish, broken off short, easily extracted; filled with trichophyton tonsurans.	5. Hairs dull, dry, brittle, easily extracted, loaded with achorion Schonleinii
6. Non-contagious.	6. Non-contagious.	6. Non-contagious.	6. Communicable by inoculation.	6. Contagious.	6. Contagious.

Prognosis.—The prognosis is always good in acute cases, but should be more or less guarded in chronic forms. Eczemas at the mucous outlets are more obstinate than those located elsewhere.

Treatment.—The diet should be regulated so as to bring in as many of the oleaginous principles as possible in place of the nitrogenous. Sweets and starches in excess must be avoided. Pork, fish, seasoned meats, pastry, pickles and stimulating drinks should be strictly forbidden. Cream should enter largely into the diet in children. In adults milk should not be taken as a beverage with meals, but alone, on an empty stomach. Mothers nursing eczematous children should abstain from taking ale, beer, wine or tea.

The local treatment consists in first allaying the acute inflammatory symptoms, if any exist. This is best done by the use of bran washes, or emollient poultices of marsh mallow, boiled starch or linseed meal.

In simple cases where there is but little inflammatory disturbance, and the discharge is the principal feature, the parts should be dusted with buckwheat flour, or with equal parts of starch and zinc oxide. When there is much itching, temporary relief is afforded by the application of cloths wrung out in hot water. Should the itching prove obstinate, a weak carbolized oil and lime water lotion, or a grindelia robusta lotion, one drachm (4.) to the ounce (32.) of water may be used.

At times oleates or ointments answer better than

either lotions or dusting powders, and this especially when, as is apt to be the case, there is outside of the discharge feature, an unnatural dryness of the skin. The benzoated oxide of zinc ointment or the oleate of zinc is the one most commonly used. Its action is protective rather than curative. It allays irritation and keeps the air from the parts, and thus aids much in performing a cure. It should be spread on the wooly side of lint and kept close to the surface. It will however be well to remember that ointments are seldom tolerated when the skin is acutely inflamed.

Too frequent washings of eczematous patients are injurious. For bathing purposes, rose water containing a little glycerine and sodium chloride should be used instead of clear water.

In sub-acute or chronic conditions a weak oleate of mercury or a white precipitate ointment, ten to thirty grains (.6 to 2.) to the ounce (32.) of vaseline, is frequently of service.

In inveterate cases, oil of white birch may be used in the form of an ointment, one-half (2.) to two drachms (8.) to the ounce (32.) of vaseline.

Ointments should as a rule be applied night and morning, and all scales should be removed, and the parts bathed before every application.

In eczema of the legs, considerable benefit may be derived from strapping the parts with Martin's elastic bandage during the day, and applying soothing dressings at night. Vulcanized India rubber gloves are of considerable value in eczema of the hands when the cuticle is thickened and hard.

The appropriate internal remedy will usually be one of the following, according to the indications:

Aconite.—In the simpler forms of eczema, and when there is much febrile disturbance. Acute cases, with stinging and pricking of the skin, in plethoric persons.

Alumina.—Hard crusts on the scalp, face and extremities. Gnawing itching, worse in the evening, not relieved by scratching. Aggravated on alternate days and from eating new potatoes. Dryness of the skin. Constipation.

AMMONIUM CARB.—Eczema in the bends of the extremities. Excoriations between the legs, and about the anus and genitals. Violent itching relieved by scratching. Aggravated by either cold applications or hot poultices. In children.

Ammonium mur.—Eczema on the face and across the loins. Intense burning, somewhat relieved by cold applications. Constipation. In fat sluggish individuals.

Anacardium.—Acute eczema on the face, neck and chest. Intense itching usually aggravated, but occasionally relieved by scratching. Redness of the skin with eruption of small vesicles. Sensitiveness to draught.

Antimonium crud.—Pustular eczema about the face and joints. Painful cracks in the corners of the mouth. Violent itching and burning, better in the open air, worse after bathing. Thick, heavy, yellow crusts upon the face. Gastric derangement with thick white coated tongue. In children who grow fat.

Antimonium tart.—Eruptions about the nose and eyes, neck and shoulders, and back of the ears. Vesicles surrounded by a red areola. Pustules, as large as peas. Itching worse in the evening, better in the open air. Eruption leaves bluish-red stains upon the face. Child wants to be carried; cries if touched. Desire for acids; aversion to milk. Rattling cough.

Apis mel.—Red and œdematous skin, with burning and stinging. Better from cold applications, worse after warm applications. Large vesicles. Urine scanty and high colored.

Argentum nit.—Eczema on the genitals. Urging to urinate. In children who eat too much sweets.

Arsenicum alb.—Eczema on the face, legs and genitals. *Intense burning of the surface.* Itching worse during the first hours of sleep. Better from external heat; worse from cold or from scratching. Dry scaly eruption with parchment-like skin. Falling out of hair in patches. Useful in chronic cases.

Arundo maurit.—Eruption on the chest, upper extremities and behind the ears. Intolerable itching, crawling sensation, especially over the loins and shoulders. In young children.

Astacus fluv.—Thick crusts on the scalp. Enlargement of the lymphatic glands. Clay colored stools.

Aurum mur.—Smarting, itching papular eruption on the lips or above the pubis. Constant desire to be out in the open air. In corpulent old people. After abuse of mercury.

Baryta carb.—Moist crusts on the scalp. Itching,

burning and pricking sensations, aggravated after washing. Falling off of the hair. Swelling and induration of the cervical glands and tonsils. Extreme sensitiveness of the scalp. In fat timid children that take cold easily.

Belladonna.—Eczema on the face with scarlet redness. Burning, itching eruption, sensitive to the touch. In teething children, with tendency to convulsions.

Borax.—Eczema on the face and scalp. Red, papulous eruption around the cheeks and chin. Excoriating secretions. Aphthous difficulties. Slight injuries suppurate. Dread of slight downward motion.

Bovista.—Grocer's itch. Moist vesicular eruption with formation of thick crusts. Eruption about the mouth and nostrils; on the thighs and bends of the knees; on the back of the hand; swelling of the upper lip; burning, itching; no relief from scratching. Symptoms worse during hot weather. General lassitude, especially about the joints. The skin of the fingers becomes dented by the use of the scissors or other instruments.

Bromine.—Eczema covering the head as with a cap, with profuse oozing of dirty, foul smelling discharge. Crawling sensation beneath the scalp, with sensitiveness to the touch. Glands of the neck hard and swollen.

Bryonia.—Eczema all over the body, *especially on the back.* Eruption slow in making its appearance. Scalp very sensitive to the touch. Aches and pains aggravated by motion. Symptoms worse from exposure to the heat of the fire.

Caladium.—Eczema on the genitals, forearm and chest. Vesicular eruption with itching and burning, worse at night. Itching and sudden violent corrosive burning, often on small spots. Attacks alternating with asthma.

CALCAREA CARB.—Thick crusts with yellow pus beneath, on the face, legs and flexures of the extremities. Burning itching, better in a warm room, aggravated by washing. Cracked skin with deep fissures. Falling off of the hair. Moist eruption behind the right ear. Hard swelling of the cervical glands. Chronic eruption, with cold feet as if damp stockings were on them. Symptoms aggravated by drinking milk. In big-bellied children with light hair and blue eyes.

Calcium sulphide.—Eczema spreading by new pimples beyond the main excoriation. Eruption worse on the scalp and behind the ears. Burning and itching of the skin after scratching. Soreness and moisture in the folds between the scrotum and thighs. Unhealthy skin, even slight injuries suppurate. Itching worse at night and on rising in the morning. Eruption very sensitive and sore to the touch.

Cantharis.—The inflammatory stage. Eruption mostly on the right side, with burning and itching. When complicated with urinary troubles.

Carbo veg.—Eczema on the legs, face and chin. Vesicles on the knees. Fine, moist eruption with burning sensation, aggravated by warmth and moisture. In cachectic individuals, accompanying dyspepsia.

Carbolic acid.—Moist vesicular eruption on the hands and all over the body. Itching better from rubbing, but leaving a burning pain.

Causticum.—Moist eruption on the nape of the neck and around the nipple. Thick crusts on the nostrils. Symptoms worse in the evening and in the open air, better from warmth. In rheumatic and gouty subjects.

Chamomilla.—Excoriations between the thighs in children and infants. Unhealthy skin, every injury suppurates. Severe itching of sweating parts. Child fretful, must be carried about.

Chelidonium.—Eczema of the scrotum and lower extremities. Heat, swelling and redness of the parts (*E. rubrum*). Bitter taste in the mouth when not eating or drinking. Pain in the hepatic region. Chronic affections of the abdominal organs.

Cicuta.—Eczema on the face with yellow scurf on the skin like dried honey. Thick, whitish scurf on the chin and upper lip with oozing. Burning itching in the parts, especially when touched.

Clematis—Moist eczema on the neck and occiput with terrible itching. Aggravated by washing in cold water, and by wet poultices. Itching temporarily relieved by scratching. Painful swelling and induration of the glands. Eruption moist during increasing, and dry during decreasing moon.

Conium.—Eczema on the face, pubes and extremities. Moist vesicles with sero-purulent discharge. Burning and itching aggravated by scratching. Glandular enlargement and induration. In aged people, and in children who are prematurely old.

Crotalus.—Vesicular eruption on the septum narium. Sour, acrid eructations. Painful retention of urine.

Croton tig.—Eczema on the face, genitals and scrotum. Swelling and redness of the face and eyelids which are covered with small vesicles. Excessive itching, better from slight scratching. Two-story pustules. Painful swelling of the glands. Painless, watery diarrhœa, gushing out forcibly. A perfect picture of all the stages of eczema in regular course.

Dulcamara.—Thick brown or yellow crusts on the temples, forehead and chin. Itching eruption aggravated by cold weather, better in warm air. Glandular swellings in the neighborhood of the eruption. Face-ache and asthma follow the disappearance of the eruption. Eruption precedes the menses.

Fluoric acid.—Eczema on the face, scalp, neck and chest. *Dry* eruption with itching and burning. Painful rhagades after washing. Brittle nails.

Graphites.—Thick crusts and a raw surface with deep rhagades. Moist eruption worse on the chin, behind the ears, on the palms of the hands and on the left side. Humid eruption with secretion of corrosive serum smelling like herring brine. Itching worse in the evening and at night. Increased sticky discharge after scratching. Skin dry, never perspires, and is inclined to crack. In blondes inclined to obesity, especially females with disposition to delayed menstruation.

Helleborus.—Small vesicles on the fingers of the right hand, humid for a long time and then covered with scurf. Sudden dropsical swelling. In weakly scrofulous children during dentition.

Hydrastis.—Eczema along the border of the hair in front. Aggravated on coming from the cold into a warm room. Oozing after washing. Constipation with hæmorrhoids.

Hypericum.—Eczema on the face and hands. Yellowish-green crusts with violent itching. Excessive itching, especially in the sacral region when undressing. The eruption is sometimes dry, aud at times fiery red. Roughness of the skin.

Iris versic.—Eczema on the face. Pustular eruption around the nose and lips, and on the cheeks. Worse in the evening and at night. Gastric and bilious derangements.

Juglans cin.—Vesicular eruption on the upper and front part of the chest with burning and itching. Violent itching over the whole body, in spots, worse when being heated from over-exertion. Stitch-like pain under the right scapula.

Kali carb.—Eczema all over the body, especially on the abdomen and around the nipples. Dry scaly spots with violent itching. Eruption dry at first but after scratching exudes a moisture. Appears in warm weather. In persons with dry skin, or who are inclined to pulmonary troubles.

Ledum.—Eczema only on covered parts. Gnawing itching of the skin, with unnatural dryness of the surface. Enlargement of the cervical glands. Adapted to rheumatic individuals and drunkards.

Lappa maj.—Eczema of the scalp extending to the face. Moist, bad smelling eruption on the heads of children. Large grayish-white crusts on the scalp with loss of hair. Swelling and suppuration of the axillary glands. Disposition to boils.

Lachesis.—Eczema on the legs. Ulcers on the lower extremities. Pricking, pulsating tearing pains. Variable appetite. Burning in the palms and soles. Often useful in women during the climacteric period.

Lycopodium.—Eczema beginning on the back of the head and extending to the face. Moist eruption with abundant foul smelling secretion. Humid eruption with fissures followed by thick crusts. Biting and itching when becoming warm and from poultices. The surface bleeds easily, after scratching. Inclined to constipation.

Mercurius.—Eczema all over the body, especially on the scalp, chin and extremities. Yellow crusts with inflamed areolæ. Intolerable itching, particularly at night or when getting warm while at work or in bed. Bleeding and smarting of the surface after scratching. Tendency to inflammation of the lymphatic glands. Patients perspire easily.

Merc. iodat.—When other remedies fail and there is a decided syphilitic taint. Swelling and induration of the glands. Troublesome itching over the whole body. All symptoms are worse at night.

MERC. PRECIP. RUBER.—Eczema of the hairy parts, and of the anus with fissures. Eczema of the umbilicus. Pustular eruption with slight itching. Oozing of pus from beneath the crusts. Glandular swellings.

Mezereum.—Honey-like scabs around the mouth. Discharges profuse, excoriate the surrounding parts. Unbearable itching increased by scratching or when undressing. Head covered with a thick, leathery crust, under which pus collects and mats the hair. Constant chilliness over the whole body.

Natrum mur.—Eczema raw and inflamed, discharging a corrosive gluey fluid. Worse along the posterior border of the hair, in the flexures of the extremities, and on the genitals. Humid eruption matting the hair. Redness and inflammation of the margins and corners of the eyelids. Great rawness and soreness of the skin, with itching and pricking.

Nitric acid.—Vesicles on the inner side of the left hand. Soreness of the feet from profuse, offensive perspiration. Dry, scaly skin. Moisture and itching in the anus. Syphilitic ulcers, after abuse of mercury. In dark complexioned old people.

NUX JUGLANS.—Burning itching vesicles upon a cracked surface, with a greenish discharge which stiffens linen. Large blood boils on the shoulders and in hepatic region. Itching worse in the evening and at night.

Oleander.—Oozing behind the ears, and on the back

of the head. Smooth shining surface covered with drops of serum Gnawing itching while undressing. Extreme sensitiveness of the skin, even the friction of the clothing causes soreness and rawness.

Petroleum.—Moist eczema on the genitals, and inside of the thighs with rawness and great itching. Profuse oozing after scratching. Excoriated running spots on the skin. The parts burn like fire. Skin of the hands cracked and rough. Eruption between the toes. Small wounds spread and ulcerate.

Piper methysticum.—Skin dry, scaly, cracked and ulcerated, especially where it is thick, as on the hands and feet.

Piper nigrum.—Eczema on the lips.

Psorinum.—Eczema disappearing in summer, but reappearing in winter. Dry and scaly eruptions with small pointed vesicles around the reddened edges. Violent itching aggravated by warmth. Dirty, greasy-looking, foul-smelling skin.

RHUS TOX.—In acute eczema. Eruption on the face and hairy parts. *Small* yellow vesicles with red areolæ. Humid eruption forming thick crusts with offensive smell. Hardness and thickening of the scrotum. Nightly itching and burning. Aggravated by changes in the weather, and by wet or cold weather.

Rhus venenata.—Fine vesicular eruption on the upper extremities. Groups of watery vesicles on the fingers. Fissures on the ends of the fingers. *Upper lip swollen and covered with vesicles.*

Sarsaparilla.—Eczema on the nose and face. Thick

scabs on the face. Scabby eruption on the nose and face, like *milk crust.* Child cries a great deal and is extremely restless.

Sepia.—Humid eruption in the flexures of the joints and behind the ears. Dry, offensive eruptions on the vertex and back of the head. Itching of the skin changing to burning when scratched. Eruption in rings during pregnancy and nursing. In dark-complexioned people.

Silicea.—Eczema on the arms and scalp. Humid eruption with greenish putrid discharge. Dry, scaly crusts. Scabs behind the ears. Itching during the day and evening, never at night. Cervical glands swollen. Offensive perspiration on the feet and genitals.

Staphysagria.—Eczema on the head and behind the ears. Eczema of the feet. Yellow, acrid, offensive moisture oozes from under the crusts. Burning and itching; scratching sometimes changes the locality of the itching. Oozing after scratching. Scalp painfully sensitive. Itching of the margins of the lids. Painful swelling of the glands. Cross words injure feelings.

Sulphur.—Eczema around the margin of the hairy scalp from ear to ear posteriorly. Crusts and pimples and easily bleeding burning and painful surface. Voluptuous itching with soreness after scratching. Genitals legs and bends of the extremities specially affected. Patient takes cold easily.

Sulphuric acid.—Moist eczema with pricking of the

skin. Scratching rarely relieves the itching, but changes its locality.

Sumbul.—Eczema on the left side of the scalp in infants.

Terebinthina.—Eczema in front of the ear in children.

Tartar emet.—Vesicular eruption about the nose, eyes, neck and shoulders. Early pustulation. Pustular eruption leaves bluish-red marks on the face. Child wants to be carried; cries if touched. Desire for acids; aversion to milk.

Thuja.—Dry scaly eruption on the head extending to the temples, eyebrows, ears and neck, with itching tingling and biting. Itching vesicles with shooting pains. Skin extremely sensitive to the touch, burning violently after scratching. Dryness of covered parts; perspiration on uncovered parts smelling like honey. In dark complexioned individuals.

Viola tricolar.—Eczema on the face. Humid eruption with intolerable nightly itching. Discharge of yellow water or pus. Swelling of the cervical glands. Verminous crusts. Urine smells like cat's urine.

Vinca minor.—Eczema on head, face, and septum of the nose. Offensive moist verminous eruption with biting itching. Yellowish discharge, forming brown crusts. Matting of the hair. Phthiriasis.

ELEPHANTIASIS.

Definition.—Elephantiasis is a chronic disease characterized by great hypertrophy of the skin and subcutaneous connective tissue, usually confined to the lower limbs and genitals.

Synonyms.—Elephantiasis arabum. Elephant leg. Barbadoes leg. Tropical big leg.

Symptomatology.—The disease is generally ushered in with a chill followed by febrile symptoms. An inflammatory swelling of the leg of an erysipelatous nature soon makes its appearance accompanied by an inflamed and painfully distended condition of the lymphatics and glands of the groin. In a few days the febrile symptoms subside, but the swelling remains, never entirely disappearing. Recurrent inflammatory attacks take place at variable intervals, which leave the leg always larger than before. Each attack is accompanied by stabbing pains in the limb, but they are more severe at the beginning than at any subsequent period of the disease. The skin is usually harder and darker than normal. In the course of a year or more, the febrile attacks cease, but the parts continue growing until they reach an enormous size.

The regions usually affected are the lower extremity of one side, and the genitals. The upper extremities and the face may likewise become involved

Etiology.—The etiology of elephantiasis is obscure. Recent investigations would, however, lead us to infer that it is due to the action of a parasite, the *filaria sanguinis*, in obstructing the lymphatics. It is supposed that the mosquito plays an important part in the development and transportation of the undeveloped filariæ.

It is more prevalent in low malarial districts and in tropical climates. Sporadic cases occur in all countries. It is endemic in the West Indies, South America, West Africa, Arabia, Southern China and Japan. It attacks males more than females and is most frequent between the ages of twenty five and sixty. It is neither hereditary nor contagious.

Prognosis.—Elephantiasis is always a grave disease, and may last a life time. It is however, more amenable to treatment now than formerly.

Treatment.—A milk diet is the best for the elephantiasis patient, and if it is a possible thing, a change of climate should be made.

Esmarch's bandage has been employed with good result, as has also prolonged compression of the main artery of the part. Excision of the sciatic nerve is recommended in some cases, and amputation as a dernier resort should not be forgotten.

Relief, and occasionally beneficial results come from the use, of hamamelis or chaulmoogra oil dressings.

MYRISTICA SEBIFERA, is the main internal remedy. *Hydrocotyle asiatica*, has been recommended, as have also Anacardium orientale and Elæis guineensis.

EPHELIS.

Definition.—Ephelis is a variety of skin discoloration, due to the deposit of pigment, excited by the action of the sun's rays.

Synonyms.—Sunburn. Tan.

Treatment.—Temporary benefit accrues from the use of local applications strong enough to cause exfoliation of the corneal cells. A one per cent solution of mercuric bichloride, and a ten per cent. solution of calcium chloride are the lotions most commonly used.

Veratrum alb., Robinia, and Kali carb. are useful internal remedies. Bufo is indicated when the face tans quickly.

EPITHELIOMA.

Definition.—Epithelioma of the skin is a malignant new growth, characterized by a tendency to increase in size, to invade the adjacent tissues, and to local recurrence after removal.

Synonyms.—Epithelial cancer. Cancroid.

Symptomatology.—Epithelial cancer may start either as a flat infiltration, a wart or other growth.

The earliest sign is often a simple crack, or little hard, pale dusky lump, which sooner or later fissures, and is then either moist, or covered with a brownish or yellowish crust.

The growth gradually increases in size and finally breaks down into superficial ulcers. The typical ulcer is roundish, split-pea sized or larger, has hard sharply defined edges, and secretes a scanty, yellow viscid fluid. This form may continue for years, running along as an apparently local affection without in any way undermining the patient's health.

It is usually met with in men, especially smokers, and selects as its favorite seat, the lower lip. On the scrotum it constitutes the *chimney sweeper's cancer.* When occurring on the upper two-thirds of the face it forms the *rodent ulcer* of English writers.

At times epithelioma commences in the form of papules, which are at first movable, but later tend to run together, and form reddish or purplish colored walnut-sized aggregatious. These eventually break down and form extensive ulcers. They are attended sooner or later by sharp lancinating pains which become almost unendurable as the disease advances. The ulcers are usually roundish, have hard everted, indurated and undermined edges, secrete an offensive pale yellow viscid fluid, and bleed easily. As the destructive process continues, tissue after tissue gives way to the invader, the lymphatic glands become enlarged and suppurate, and the patient ultimately succumbs from exhaustion. This form attacks by preference the mucous membrane and cheeks, but may appear on any part of the body. Its course may be either slow or rapid, and when left to itself it usually destroys life in from two to five years.

Occasionally epithelial cancer develops as wart-like growths or cauliflower excrescences that vary in size from a split pea to a hazel-nut, and ultimately break down, forming irregularly shaped granulating, easily bleeding excavations, which slowly run the course of other epitheliomatous ulcers.

Etiology.—The etiology of epithelioma is obscure. The disease rarely occurs before middle life.

Pathology.—The disease consists of a perverted growth of the epithelial elements of the skin.

Diagnosis.—It may be confounded with syphilis and lupus vulgaris. The history of the cases, however, are different. Syphilitic formations are always more rapidly developed than epitheliomatous. The ulcers of syphilis are generally multiple, have an abundant secretion, and are devoid of pain, while those of epithelioma are usually single, with scanty secretion, and severe lancinating pain.

Lupus vulgaris is commonly a disease of childhood; epithelioma is an affection of middle life. The discharge from the epitheliomatous ulcer is generally offensive, while that from lupus is not.

Prognosis.—In the early stages the disease may generally be cured. Old, extensive, or neglected cases are apt to prove fatal.

Treatment.—The growth should be removed by the knife, the galvano-caustic, or what is perhaps preferable, Marsden's arsenical mucilage. Marsden's mucilage consists of arsenious acid, two drachms (8.) and mucilage of gum acacia, one drachm (4.) mixed together into a thick paste, with a few drops of water. It is to be spread upon the part, after the removal of the crusts, and allowed to dry on. A little lint or cotton batting should be pressed on to the part overlapping the paste about half an inch. After from six to twelve hours the parts should be poulticed with bread and milk poultices renewed every two hours, until the slough separates from the healthy tissues. The piece of lint or cotton saturated with the paste should be left adherent as long as possible. Not more than one square inch of surface should be covered with the paste at one time. At times a second application is required.

The *chromium chloride* used as a paint has been recommended, and hydrastis dressings may occasionally be used with benefit.

THUJA is the principal internal remedy. Favorable mention may be made of *Sepia*, *Arsenicum alb.*, Condurango, Lapis alba, and Needham's extract of red clover blossom.

ERYTHEMA.

Definition.—Though strictly a symptom, meaning simple redness or hyperæmia, and occurring in the course of a variety of diseases, erythema is by common consent, the name given to an inflammation of the skin characterized by the appearance of macules, papules or tubercles, attended by more or less itching and burning.

Symptomatology.—The first symptom may be the appearance of one or more erythematous or slightly reddened patches, of variable size and shape. They may be circular in form, the redness gradually disappearing in the center and extending at the periphery, (E. annulare.) Several of the circles may run together and by blending in segments, give to the redness a serpentine aspect, (E. gyratum.) Occasionally variegated concentric rings may be formed (E. iris,) but generally the disease appears in the form of distinct papules, (E. papulatum,) or tubercles, (E. tuberculatum,) of variable size and shape, having a bluish color and lasting about a week. All these varied forms of manifestation are but stages of one and the same process, and not separate affections.

Erythema usually runs an acute course, and appears symmetrically. It attacks by preference the backs of the hands and feet, the arms, the legs, and the forehead. It is mostly an affection of children, and young people. It attacks females more than males, and prevails in the spring and fall. Individuals who are troubled with it one year, are apt to have it again at the same time in succeeding years. When occurring on the fingers it closely resembles chilblains. It may be commonly known by its superficial and protean character, and its symmetrical distribution.

Treatment.—When there is much itching and burning either a carbolic acid or veratrum viride lotion may be used. When the opposing surfaces are much inflamed they may be protected by dusting with buckwheat powder, or equal parts of starch and zinc oxide.

The internal remedies are:

ACONITE.—Erythema excited by the action of the sun's rays.

Æthusa.—Appearance and disappearance of reddish-blue spots on the trunk and left leg. General malaise.

Ailanthus.—Irregular spots of capillary congestion. Dark almost livid eruption on the forehead.

ARSENICUM IODIDE.—Erythema especially of the face.

BELLADONNA.—Inflamed red patches. *Irregularly* shaped scarlet spots over the body. More on face and upper part of body.

Berberis.—Mottled spots as after a bruise on the right shoulder, left humerus, back of the hand and wrist.

Bryonia.—*Red round hot spots* on the malar bone, as large as peas.

Cadmium sulph.—Red spots on the extremities.

CHELIDONIUM MAJ.—Round red spots, size of a half dollar, accompanied with burning pain, on anterior surface of the forearms and face, disappearing in a few hours.

CHLORAL HYDRATE.—Bright red or bluish erythema over the whole body, permanent under pressure, mottled with livid patches and deep red spots. Pruritus of the whole skin.

Crocus sat.—Circumscribed red spots on the face, which burn.

Condurango.—Erythematous blotches on the face and arms.

Gelsemium.—Papulous eruption on the face resembling measles.

Gossypium.—Round little spots with pale red circles around the knee caps and over the shin bones, which itch very much.

LACTIC ACID.—Several bright red blotches on the anterior surface of the leg, with slight burning and no itching. Relieved by cold. Eruption brightest at 8 A. M.

Laurocerasus.—Erythematous patches, terminating in dark red purple spots.

Mercurius sol.—Light red patches on the forearm

and inner side of the thighs. Itching changed to burning by scratching.

MEZEREUM.—Erythema on the legs in old people.

NUX VOM.—Pimples on the face with itching burning after drinking wine or alcoholic liquors.

Phytolacca.—Painful erythematous blotches of a pale red color.

Pulsatilla nut.—Erythema of the scalp. Dark blue or red eruption on the legs and ankles.

Rhus tox.—Ridges on the lower limbs.

Sabadilla.—Red streaks on the arms. Worse from cold.

USTILAGO.—Fine eruption of a deep red color, about the size of a pin's head, appearing on any part of the body after scratching. On the neck it takes a circular form.

ERYTHEMA NODOSUM.

Definition.—*See* Dermatitis contusiformis.

ERYSIPELAS.

Definition.—Erysipelas is an acute inflammatory disease of the skin, more commonly of the head and face, characterized by heat, pain, redness and swelling, and a tendency to the formation of vesicles, accompanied with more or less febrile disturbance.

Synonym.—St. Anthony's fire.

Symptomatology.—The disease usually begins with a feeling of chilliness, headache, loss of appetite and pain in the lumbar region. Frequently there is gastric distress with nausea and vomiting. The tongue becomes furred and at times dry. The pulse is rapid and the temperature rises often to 105° F. or 106° F. in some cases it reaches 108° F.

The eruption is first noticed in the form of a red, shining and slightly swollen roundish patch, from which it spreads rapidly until a large portion of surface becomes involved. The parts are somewhat sensitive to the touch, and the patient complains of pain with burning and itching sensations. The redness fades temporarily under pressure to a yellowish-white. As the disease extends, the skin becomes of a darker red color, and the swelling increases. At times owing to the rapid exudation of serum beneath the epidermis, vesicles or bullæ are formed.

In certain cases the inflammation moves from place to place, and is of short duration in each locality. This form is called *erysipelas migrans*, migratory or wandering erysipelas.

In moderate cases the inflammation usually reaches its maximum within a week. The temperature then begins to fall, the redness fades, the swelling gradually subsides, and the cuticle over the part desquamates. If the inflammation has invaded the hairy parts, the hairs are apt to fall when recovery ensues.

In severe cases the febrile, nervous, and other symptoms are grave, and death may result from complications, shock, exhaustion or pyæmia.

Surgical accidents aside, the face is the commonest seat of erysipelas. All other regions may however, be invaded. When the disease attacks the face it nearly always begins at the side of the nose near the angle of the eye.

Etiology.—The etiology of erysipelas remains as yet an uncertainty. At times it seems to be the result of a contagion, and it then assumes a severe form. Not infrequently it arises from mild or severe traumatism. The incautious use of Arnica sometimes occasions an attack. A micro-organism has been recently discovered in the blood in well marked cases.

Erysipelas leaves a very great susceptibility to renewed attacks.

Diagnosis.—Erysipelas is to be distinguished from, erythema, zoster, eczema and scarlet fever. As a rule it is readily differentiated by the constitutional symptoms and the character of the lesions.

Prognosis.—In the majority of cases the disease terminates favorably. The prognosis should, however, be guarded when the very young, the aged, the cachectic or the intemperate are attacked. Facial erysipelas is the most serious.

Treatment.—If there is considerable heat or irritability of the skin the surface may be powdered with rye or buckwheat flour, and if there is much inflammatory swelling a veratrum viride lotion may be employed. When the erysipelatous blush presents a distinctly circumscribed outline the extension of the disease is ofttimes limited by the application of the tincture of iodine with a camel's hair brush over a peripheral zone an inch in width.

Rhus is the principal internal remedy for vesicular

erysipelas, *Bell.* for non-vesicular erysipelas, *Apis* when there is much swelling, and *Graphites* or *Pulsatilla* for wandering erysipelas.

Other remedies may be indicated as follows:

Aconite.—In simple erysipelas with febrile disturbance.

Apis.—Erysipelas of the face, and scalp with œdematous swelling of the eyelids. Stinging burning, pricking pains in the skin. The eruption passes from right to left and is rather pale than deep red.

Arnica.—Erysipelas with tendency to formation of bullæ. Extreme tenderness and painfulness on pressure.

Arsenicum.—Erysipelas with gangrenous tendency. Excessive general prostration.

Belladonna.—Bright-red non-vesicular swelling especially of the right side. Intense fever, the skin imparts a burning sensation to the hand. Brain symptoms prominent. Tendency of the inflammation to spread in streaks.

Borax.—Simple erysipelas of the left side of the face. Sensation as if covered by cobwebs.

Bryonia.—Erysipelas around the joints with drawing tearing pains increased by motion.

Cantharis.—Erysipelas with fine burning stinging pains. Large blisters. The eruption begins on the nose and spreads to the cheeks, more to the right side. Urinary complications. After abuse of Arnica.

Cuprum.—Tendency to metastasis to the brain. Violent brain symptoms.

Euphorbium.—Erysipelas of the head and face with

digging, boring and gnawing pains, followed when ameliorated by creeping and itching of the part. Considerable swelling. Small vesicles discharging a yellowish fluid.

Graphites.—Tendency to repeated attacks, passing from right to left. Erysipelas of the head and face with burning, tingling pains. Swelling and induration of the lymphatics and glands.

Hydrastis.—Erysipelas wandering from left side of nose to right over entire face and scalp. Intense pain with creeping chills in small of back. Great restlessness. Urinary suppression. Used both internally and locally.

Lachesis.— Erysipelas especially on the left side. The eruption has a purplish, leaden hue. Cerebral symptoms, worse from noon until midnight. Delirium on closing the eyes.

Ledum.—Erysipelas from bites of insects.

Nux vom.—Cardialgia. Burning itching all over the skin, worse in the evening. Bright red swelling of the knees and feet with intense pain.

Phos. acid.—Erysipelas produced by traumatism, where the periosteum is affected.

Pulsatilla.—Wandering erysipelas. Erysipelas of the ears. Indigestion after disappearance of eruption.

Rhus.—Vesicular erysipelas with swelling and shining redness. The eruption spreads from left to right. Burning and itching worse at night. Extreme restlessness. Pain in back and limbs, worse during rest. Œdema with dark bluish redness of the parts. Typhoid symptoms.

Sulphur.—Migratory erysipelas with intense itching.

Veratrum vir.—Vesicular erysipelas, accompained by high fever and marked cerebral disturbance. Tendency to convulsions.

FAVUS.

Definition.—See Tinea favosa.

FIBROMA.

Definition.—Fibroma is characterized by sessile or pedunculated outgrowths from the connective tissue, generally club-shaped, and varying in size from a pea to a large pear.

Synonym.—Polypus of the skin.

Symptomatology.—The polypi or tumors are as a rule unattended with pain. They may either remain stationary or grow to a considerable size. In consistence the smaller are usually soft, and the larger more elastic and fibrous. When large they are apt to take on ulceration.

Treatment.—The larger tumors may be removed by the knife, the galvano-caustic, or the elastic ligature. The smaller ones gradually disappear under the local use of the acid nitrate of mercury.

The *arseniate of calcarea* and *lycopodium* are the principal internal remedies.

FISH-SKIN DISEASE.

Definition.—See Ichthyosis.

FRAMBŒSIA.

Definition.—Frambœsia is an endemic contagious

disease, characterized by variously sized reddish papules, tubercles and tumors, in all stages of development.

Synonyms.—Yaws. Endemic verrugas.

Symptomatology.—The eruptions start as pin-head sized points and gradually increase in size so as to resemble in their different stages of development, first a currant, then a raspberry, and lastly a cherry. Later on in their course they are apt to break down and ulcerate, pouring out a thin yellowish offensive discharge.

The disease is almost wholly confined to tropical climates, and principally met with among the colored races. It rarely occurs twice in the same individual. It attacks mostly the face and genitals, and occasionally the upper and lower extremities. It is endemic in the West Indies and in South America and Africa.

Treatment.—Cleanliness, nourishing diet and a well regulated hygiene are highly important.

The local treatment consists in using a jatropha lotion having the prepared strength of from one drachm (4.) to two drachms (8.) of jatropha tincture to the ounce (32.) of distilled water, or else a week nitrate of mercury ointment.

The *iodides* of *mercury* and *potassium* are the most efficacious internal remedies.

FURUNCLE.

Definition.—Furuncle is an acute localized inflammation of the skin and connective tissue, varying in size from a small pea to a hickory-nut, having an indurated and inflamed base, and usually terminating in suppuration and the formation of a "core".

Synonym.—Boil.

Symptomatology.—The boil commences as a small roundish, inflamed spot, tender to the touch, and surrounded by a bright red areola, which changes to purple as the disease advances. It gradually increases in size, becomes more and more sensitive to the touch, and the pain which is usually of a throbbing nature increases in intensity.

After running an increasingly painful course of five or six days, the rounded swelling suppurates and throws out a central slough called a "core". At times the suppurative stage is scarcely reached, and no core forms. It is then termed a "blind" boil. After the discharge, the pain, redness and inflammatory symptoms quickly subside, the patient feels relieved, and unless there are more to follow, his troubles are over. Generally, however, this is but a fore-taste of things to come, and the end is not yet.

Furuncles may make their appearance on any part of the body, but attack by preference, the face, back and gluteal region, and may start either in the hair follicles, sebaceous glands or surrounding cellular tissue. They are usually dependent upon disordered blood-states, or depraved conditions of system, and are sometimes epidemic. They are more common at the extremes of life, but may occur at any age.

Treatment.—Patients should be well hygiened and given a good wholesome diet. In debilitated states the free use of porter may eradicate the tendency to boils. Brewers' yeast, in tablespoonful doses between meals, has the reputation of being a preventive. A ten per cent muriate of lime lotion well rubbed on the parts when boils threaten, sometimes occasions their abortion. When a boil is tense and hard, the best local treatment consists in applying hot, limited flax seed meal or tomato poultices. Poultices should not be continued after the boil opens, as if too long used they rather encourage the formation of new boils. After the boil is fully matured if it has not already opened, it may be incised and the contents evacuated. Gelsemium or lappa cerate is a good after dressing.

The appropriate internal remedy will usually be one of the following:

Absinthium.—Eruption of furuncles over the whole body.

Æthusa.—Painful boil on the small of the back. Hepatic derangement. Intolerance of milk. In children during dentition.

Ammonium carb.—Boils on the cheeks and around the ear. In scrofulous children, and in old people.

ANTIMONIUM CRUD.—Boils on the perineum. Burning pain for some distance around. Gastric derangement.

Arnica.—Many small boils on the face. Eructations bitter and like rotten eggs. General lassitude.

Apis mel.—Boils on the pubis. Burning, stinging pains. Great sensitiveness to touch and pressure.

BELLADONNA.—In early stage, if boil is inflamed and

painful. Red, hot, shining swelling. Boils on the shoulders every spring. After measles.

Bellis per.—Boils beginning as slight pimples, and increasing to large dark colored swellings, with aching pain. Mostly on the *neck* and lower jaw.

Berberis vulg.—Hastens suppuration in boils, and prevents their recurrence.

Bromine.—Boils on the arms and face. In light-haired, blue-eyed persons.

Cadmium sulph.—Boils on the nose and buttocks.

Calcarea carb.—Boils on the forearms and hands, with lancinating pains. Cramps in the arms. Glandular swellings. In scrofulous individuals.

Calcarea mur.—As a preventive.

Calcium sulphide.—When boils mature slowly. Violent throbbing gathering pain. Stinging soreness. After injuries.

Carbo animalis.—Boils at the anus. Burning, tearing pain. In scrofulous subjects.

Cina.—Boils on the head and face in children. Child is very fretful; bores in the nose with the fingers. Burning heat of the face with glowing redness of the cheeks.

Gelsemium.—Large boils on the face and neck. Great muscular prostration. Sleeplessness from nervous irritation. Dizziness and blurred vision. Heat of face and head.

Kalmia lat.—Red inflamed spots like incipient boils.

Lappa maj.—Boils on the face, eyelids and all over.

Ledum.—Boils on the forehead. Itching, pricking tearing pains worse in the evening before midnight. After mosquito stings. In drunkards.

Lycopodium.—Boils on the nates. Periodical boils. Aggravated by warm, wet poultices. After excessive wine drinking.

Manganum.—Small boils. Every injury tends to suppurate.

Magnesia mur.—Boils on the nose which suppurate in twenty-four hours. Boils on the false ribs. Menstrual derangements. Diarrhœa in children.

Merc. sol.—Boils on the ankles. Coldness of the hands and feet. Fœtid ulcers on the legs, with gnawing itching. Shooting tensive pains, worse at night.

Natrum carb.—Boils behind the ears. Ulcers on the heel. Burning in the feet when walking. Sour eructations.

Nitric acid.—Numerous large boils on the scapulæ nape of the neck, nates, thighs and legs. Tensive pains worse in the evening and at night. Aggravated by drinking milk.

Nitrum.—Boils on the thumb.

Nux juglans.—Boils on the right arm. Indurated boils. Blood boils. Violent itching and burning.

Nux vom.—Boils on the knees. Gastric derangement. Constipation.

Phosphoric acid.—Boils in the axillæ, and on the nates. Burning, stinging pain. Skin feels sore all over. In young people who grow rapidly.

Phytolacca.—Boils on the back.

RHUS RAD.—Boils on the face which do not mature. Blind boils.

Silicea.—Boils on the posterior portion of the thighs, and on the calves. Disposition to boils. Constipation. Mal-assimilation.

Stramonium.—Boils on the feet. Coldness of the limbs in children.

SULPHUR.—Boils in the ear. Stinging itching with smarting after scratching; after suppressed menstruation. Disposition to boils.

Zincum ox.—Boils on the abdomen, aggravated by use of wine. Worse before and during menstruation. Constipation.

GROCER'S ITCH.

Definition.—Grocer's itch is an inflammation of the skin due to the irritant action of sugar. See Eczema.

GUINEA-WORM DISEASE.

Symptomatology.—Guinea-worm disease is a common affection in tropical climates, due to the parasite known as the *filaria medinensis.* The young worm when quite small bores its way into the skin, generally of one of the lower extremities, and there takes up its abode. It remains in a quiescent state in the connective tissue for months, until it attains the length of three or six decimeters. More or less local irritation is by this time caused by its presence, and generally a pointed tumor surmounted by a bleb forms, accompanied by swelling and pain, which sooner or later breaks, showing the worm in situ. There is as a rule only one worm to each tumor.

Treatment.—The treatment consists in removing the worm two or three centimeters at a time, care being taken not to break it, and winding it around a quill until all is removed. The sore may then be dressed as an ordinary ulcer. Arsenicum alb. or mercurius may be useful as an internal remedy.

HERPES.

Definition.—Herpes is an acute inflammation of the skin, characterized by the appearance of groups of vesicles having reddened, slightly inflamed bases, and situated for the most part on the face and genitals.

Symptomatology.—The disease is generally preceded by malaise and slight febrile symptoms. A feeling of heat and distress, with redness and swelling, is usually present at the outbreak of the eruption, but gradually declines after its appearance. The vesicles appear in clusters, and are commonly bilateral. They are larger than those of eczema, but smaller than those of zoster. On the third day, as a rule, they either rupture or commence drying up, to form thin scales which drop off in a day or two, leaving discolorations which soon disappear. Herpes may occur on any part of the face or genitals, but is commonly encountered about the end of the lips, the prepuce, labia and mons veneris.

It tends to recur more on the male genitals than on the female, and is apt to be mistaken for chancroid.

It is chiefly excited by cold, and may be symptomatic, as in the herpetic patches, called "cold sores," that appear on the lip and face in catarrh and pneumonia, and the crisis of fevers.

Occasionally it appears about the seventh month of pregnancy in the form of successive crops of vesicles, beginning upon the extremities and attended with excessive itching (*H. gestationis*). The eruption frequently lasts until delivery, and then suddenly disappears. Sometimes it re-appears the third day after parturition.

At times the disease is characterized by the occurrence of vesicles in circles about a central one (*H. iris*).

Treatment.—The local treatment consists in the use of camphor cerate, calendula jelly or cologne water.

The internal remedies are:

ACONITE.—In the earlier stages with catarrhal fever.

Agnus castus.—Herpes on the cheeks with gnawing itching, worse from getting wet.

Alnus rubra.—Chronic herpes.

ARS. ALB.—Red herpetic skin around the mouth, with *burning*, worse from scratching and after midnight. Herpes iris.

Apis mel.—Large confluent vesicles. Burning *stinging* pains. Vesicular eruption on the lips. Cold sores.

Aurum mur.—Herpes on the prepuce and vulva. Herpes accompanied by intolerable itching.

BUFO.—Herpetic eruption after a cold.

Causticum.—Burning vesicles under the prepuce which become suppurating ulcers. Burning vesicles on the face which, when touched, exude a corrosive water, afterward they dry up to a scurf.

CALCIUM SULPHIDE.—Herpes which tends to recur.

Herpes on the prepuce, exceedingly sensitive to the touch. Small ulcers form around the large one. Unhealthy suppurating skin, after mercurial poisoning.

Cantharis.—Large, burning painful blisters with erysipelatous inflammation of the parts. Burning, tearing ulcerative pains. Worse on the right side. Urinary complications.

Clematis.—Itching blisters on the lower lip. Gnawing itching not relieved by scratching. Worse during increasing, better during decreasing moon.

Graphites.—Herpes in females with scanty menstruation. Burning blisters on the lower side and tip of the tongue. Dryness of the skin.

Hamamelis.—Herpes on the nose. Profuse epistaxis.

Helleborus nig.—White vesicles on the lips. Aphthæ in the mouth. In scrofulous children.

KALI BICH.—Herpes after taking cold. Fluent coryza. All the secretions are of a stringy and ropy character.

MERCURIUS SOL.—Herpes on the prepuce with a tendency to suppuration. Ulcers on the glans. Itching of the genitals.

Moschus.—Herpes with excessive burning, in hysterical subjects. Menstruation too early and too profuse.

NATRUM MUR.—Herpes occurring during fevers. Eruption on the lips and flexures of the joints. Vesicles on the tongue. Itching and pricking in the skin.

Petroleum.—Herpes on the perineum and genitals. Itching worse in the open air.

RHUS TOX.—Herpes upon the hairy parts with burning and stinging. Itching worse after scratching. Rheumatic pains with great weariness.

SEPIA.—Herpetic eruptions around the lips. Herpes during pregnancy. Circular form of eruption.

Sulphur.—Herpes about the mouth and nose with itching and burning. Itching aggravated by warmth. Hot palms and soles.

SARSAPARILLA.—Herpes on the prepuce. After abuse of mercury.

Upas.—Herpetic eruption on the upper lip, on the left side.

HIRSUTIES.

Definition.—Hirsuties is an abnormal development of hair and may be either congenital or acquired.

Synonyms.—Polytrichia. Hypertrichosis. Trichauxis. Augmented hairy growth.

Symptomatology.—Congenital hirsuties is a rare deformity, although it is a not uncommon occurrence for infants at birth to display long hairs on hairy parts, which soon fall and are replaced by shorter hairs. At times the excessive growth covers the whole surface as in so-called "hairy men." And again it may be localized to small areas as on moles.

Acquired hirsuties occurs mostly in women, upon parts generally covered with lanugo or downy hairs, such as the upper lip, chin, cheeks and arms. Occasionally in men, this hypertrophy affects the hairs of the scalp or head, which acquire enormous vigor and length.

Hirsuties is more common in dark than in ligh complexioned persons. It in no way affects the general health, and is troublesome only in consequence of the disfigurement it occasions.

Etiology.—The causes of hypertrophy of the hairs is enshrouded in mystery. Not uncommonly in women it is associated with uterine or ovarian disease.

Treatment.—The treatment is principally local, and consists in the destruction of the individual hair follicles. This may be accomplished by epilation and the introduction of a straight glover's needle dipped in carbolic acid into each follicle and rotating it several times. Piffard's improved needle holder with lens attachment affords more accurate penetration of the follicle than can be attained by the use of the simple needle. Electrolysis may also be employed with advantage. The needle is connected with the negative pole of a galvanic battery—using from six to eight cells—and inserted into the follicle, the circuit is then closed by the patient touching the positive electrode with the hand. In about thirty seconds the follicle will be destroyed with the formation of a foam around it, and the hair may be readily removed.

Depilatory powders though often used are not to be relied upon. The sulphide of barium depilatory powder, prepared by mixing two drachms (8.) of sulphide of barium, three drachms (12.) of oxide of zinc, and three drachms (12.) of amylum, is the best. It may be mixed with water and put on as a paste, allowed to remain five or ten minutes and then scraped off, and the surface anointed with cosmoline.

Lycopodium has been recommended as an internal remedy.

HYDROA.

Definition.—Hydroa is a disease characterized by the eruption of isolated vesicles which tend to recur.

Symptomatology.—As a skin affection it stands midway between herpes and pemphigus, and is mostly a reflex of excited nerve states. It starts as little papules which ultimately become vesicles, and is usually preceded and accompanied by more or less pruritus. It attacks by preference the face, extensor surfaces of the limbs, and the genitals, is generally symmetrically developed, and runs its course in two or three weeks.

Treatment.—The water of the Salzburg springs, Austria, has considerable reputation in curing skin affections, and notably hydroa.

POTASSIUM IODIDE, KREASOTE and Magnesia carb are the principal remedies.

HYDRO-ADENITIS.

Definition.—Hydro-adenitis is an inflammation of the perspiratory follicles and adjacent connective tissue, ordinarily terminating in suppuration.

Symptomatology.—It may occur on any part of the body except the soles of the feet, but is most common in the axillæ, around the nipple, and on the perineum. It is usually an acute affection, and commences by the formation of one or more bright red and inflamed pea-sized swellings.

In a few days suppuration takes place, and a little

abscess is formed which eventually ruptures, and terminates the disease. This affection has generally been described as a variety of furuncle, but it differs from it in being deeper seated, and in being devoid of a "core."

Treatment.—Hot fomentations may be used to allay the inflammation.

PHOSPHORIC ACID is the internal remedy for hydro-adenitis in the axillæ.

Phosphorus, when around the nipples, and Nitric acid when on the perineum.

HYPERÆSTHESIA.

Definition.—Hyperæsthesia, by which is meant an increased sensibility of the skin, is commonly the result of some functional or organic derangement of the nervous system.

HYPERIDROSIS.

Definition.—Hyperidrosis is a functional disorder of the sweat glands, characterized by excessive sweating.

Synonyms.—Ephidrosis. Excessive sweating.

Symptomatology.—It may be either general or local, symmetrical or unilateral. In the general form it occurs quite frequently in connection with various febrile disorders, and in such diseases as pneumonia, rheumatism and tuberculosis. In disturbances of the nervous system it is often unilateral.

The local form is most common on the head, hands, feet, and genitals. Hyperidrosis occurs in the young and the old alike, and affects females as well as males. Flat-footed people are especially obnoxious to it. In its causation faulty innervation play an important part.

The patient complains of tenderness with more or less burning. The sole and region of the toes, if the foot is the part affected, present a reddish or pinkish appearance.

Prognosis.—The prognosis should always be guarded, as many cases prove intractable.

Treatment.—Water should be applied to the parts as seldom as possible, and in bathing, the juniper tar soap is the best to use. Dusting powders of zinc oxide and starch or French chalk and starch are often serviceable. In some cases the best results are obtained from foot baths of infusion of white oak bark.

The commonly indicated internal remedies in hyperidrosis are:

BAPTISIA—In critical sweats. Frequent sweat from the small of the back in all directions.

BELLADONNA.—Sweat on covered parts. Sweat during sleep. Suddenly occurring and suddenly disappearing sweat.

Bryonia.—Sweat in short spells and only on single parts. Oppressive drawing in the head as the sweating subsides.

CALCAREA CARB.—Sweating from the least exercise. Cold clammy sweat on the legs at night. Foot sweat makes the foot sore. The feet feel cold and damp.

Chamomilla.—Excessive sweating in women after confinement..

CINCHONA.—Exhausting night sweats. Partial cold sweat on the face and all over the body with thirst.

Cocculus.—Morning sweat principally on the chest.

Conium.—Sweats on falling asleep. Night and morning sweat with smarting of the skin.

Crocus.—Sweat on the lower half of the body.

Ferrum.—Profuse long lasting sweat. Clammy debilitating sweat. In anæmic persons.

Graphites.—Sweat from the slightest motion. The feet sweat profusely, and there is soreness between the toes after walking.

JABORANDI.—Copious sweating and salivation. Profuse secretion from most of the glandular structures of the body.

Kali carb.—Sweat mostly on the upper part of the body, especially after eating.

LACTIC ACID.—Profuse inoffensive sweating of the feet.

Nux vom.—Sweat upon the upper half of the body. Sour morning sweat upon the right side.

Phosphorus.—Sweat mostly on the head, hands and feet. Profuse night sweat during sleep.

Phosphoric acid.—Sweat on the occiput and neck with sleepiness and thirst.

Polyporus off.—(In five grain doses) for the excessive sweats of consumptives.

Pulsatilla.—Left sided sweat. Sweat only on the face and head.

Sambucus.—Profuse weakening sweat, especially when awake. Dry heat during sleep.

SELENIUM.—Profuse sweats in the arm pits and on the genitals. Sweat stains the linen yellow or white, and stiffens it. Sweat on the anterior surface of the body.

Sepia.—Sweat on the posterior surface of the body. Offensive foot sweat causing soreness between the toes.

Silicea.—Sweat about the head in large bellied children. Worse with the change of the moon.

Sulphuric acid.—Excessive sweating. Better from drinking wine.

Thuja.—Sweat only on uncovered parts. Suppressed foot sweat.

Veratrum alb.—Cold, clammy sweat staining the linen yellow. Worse on the forehead.

ICHTHYOSIS.

Definition.—Ichthyosis is a congenital chronic disease of the skin, characterized by increased growth of the papillary layer with dryness, roughness and general scaliness.

Synonym.—Fish-skin disease.

Symptomatology.—The mildest form of this affection, occurs in children of two years and upwards, and presents a dry harsh dirty looking skin, covered with a variable amount of furfuraceous scales (*Xeroderma.*)

In severer cases, or when further developed the papillæ become enlarged, the discoloration grows more marked, and the epidermal scales are lozenge-shaped, and are separated by numerous lines and fissures (*I. simplex.*) In more extreme cases still, the scales form dry, hard, brittle plates of a yellowish or greenish hue, separated by white intervening lines, which mark the natural furrows of the skin. (*These plates never overlap one another.*) At times the scales become heaped up into black papillary horny projections. To this extreme condition the term *ichthyosis hystrix* has been applied, from its fancied resemblance to the quills of a porcupine.

In ichthyosis the whole surface of the body is usually more or less involved, and the front of the knees especially so. The face and flexures of the elbows and knees, however, generally escape. There is always attending the disease a characteristic diminution or absence of perspiration.

It is apt to be much worse in the winter time, so that the face and hands become extensively chapped and painful.

Diagnosis.—The diagnosis is generally easy, as pityriasis is the only disease to which it bears any resemblance. In pityriasis it should be remembered, the skin is more or less hyperæmic, while in ichthyosis it is not. The scales in pityriasis are "branny" and fall off readily while those of ichthyosis resemble "fish-scales" and are more adherent.

Prognosis.—Ichthyosis though very intractable, seldom proves fatal.

Treatment.—A generous diet should be allowed the patient, and cod liver oil should be a standing order.

After every full bath—the Turkish bath being the

best—the body should be anointed with either olive, chaulmoogra or cod liver oil, well rubbed in.

An infusion of quillaya saponaria bark sometimes works well as a local application.

ARSENICUM IODIDE is the principal internal remedy.

Others may be indicated as follows :

ARSENICUM IODIDE.—Dry scaly skin. Itching and burning. In scrofulous subjects with swelling of the lymphatic glands.

Clematis.—When there are fine scales with some itching, worse when getting warm in bed. Painful swelling and induration of the glands. Eruption changes character with the changes of the moon.

Graphites.—Skin dry and inclined to crack. Unhealthy skin ; every injury tends to ulceration. Thick and crippled toe nails. Extremities go to sleep. Itching of the genitals.

Iodine.—The skin has a brown dingy color. Ravenous hunger. Swelling and distension of the abdomen. Emaciation in dark complexioned, scrofulous children.

Mercurius.—Dirty, yellow color of the skin. Itching, worse at night when warm in bed. Dry, scaly spots. In syphilitic and scrofulous subjects.

Natrum carb.—Skin of the whole body becomes dry, rough and cracked here and there. Frequent empty or sour eructations. Great prostration.

PHOSPHORUS.—Skin is dry and wrinkled. Skin of hands is rough and dry. Pains in the chest. Desire for acids and spicy foods. Falling of the hair. Great indisposition. In tall, slender people.

Potassium iodide.—Skin dried up. Rough, like hog skin. Sensitive swelling of the thyroid gland. Œdematous infiltration of the tissues. After mercury or syphilis.

PLUMBUM.—Dry skin. Absolute lack of perspiration. Obstinate constipation. Paralytic weakness of the limbs.

THUJA.—Dirty gray cadaverous looking skin. Wart-shaped excrescences. Brittle or soft nails. Lymphatic temperament.

IMPETIGO CONTAGIOSA.

Definition.—Impetigo contagiosa is an acute inflammatory contagious affection, occurring mostly in children, and characterized by the presence of one or more discrete vesicles or vesico-pustules, generally umbilicated, varying in size from a split pea to a hazel-nut, and followed by flat, large straw-colored, usually fungoid, crusts.

Symptomatology.—This disease is usually ushered in by a period preceding the eruption, characterized by more or less fever and malaise. After two or three days this stage is followed by crops of small vesicles, which gradually develop into vesico-pustules and pustules.

The vesicles which are at first small, grow rapidly and may at maturity have reached the size of even a split pea or a hazel-nut. They are generally umbilicated and contain a lymph-like fluid with granular and subsequently pus cells. Red areolæ more or less extensive usually surround them.

In five or six days after their first appearance, their fluid contents begin to dry up, and eventually form flat-shaped, *straw-colored* scabs about the size of split peas or hazel-nuts, *looking as if stuck on.*

In mild cases the eruption may be confined to the skin of the forehead and cheeks, its most usual seat, but quite frequently it extends to the arms and head, and may implicate the mucous membrane of the eyes, mouth and nasal cavity.

Impetigo contagiosa was first described by Tilbury Fox in 1864. It generally occurs in children of the poorer classes, though the rich are not exempt. It may be epidemic but is mostly sporadic, and is both contagious and auto-inoculable. It tends to run a definite course and usually lasts from one to two weeks. At the Central Homœopathic Dispensary of this city it constitutes about one per cent. of all skin affections. Its most frequent cause is vaccination.

It can hardly be considered a parasitic affection, for although a fungus similar to that observed in the vaccine crust has been seen in the scabs of this disease, none have as yet been found in the fluid of the vesicle, or vesico-pustule.

Diagnosis.—By bearing in mind that this affection occurs mostly in children and frequently in those who are perfectly healthy, that it is preceded by more or less febrile disturbance, consists of isolated vesicles usually umbilicated, of split-pea size or larger, seated mostly in the face, following generally in the wake of vaccination, and presenting scabs having the characteristic appearance as if "stuck on," it can hardly be mistaken for any of the other forms of cutaneous trouble. The diseases with which it is most liable to be confounded are eczema and varicella. It may be distinguished from the former by the fact that the children attacked are usually healthy, while those of eczema are not; that the scabs are light yellow, flat and "look as if stuck on," while those of eczema are greenish yellow and adherent; that it is generally confined to the face and upper extremities, while eczema may attack any part of the body.

From varicella it may be known by the smaller vesicles and different crusts of the latter, together with the almost constant constitutional disturbance and the appearance of vesicles on all parts of the body.

Treatment.—The patient should be well nourished, and if there is much inflammation around the vesicles, the soothing applications spoken of in eczema should be used. White precipitate cerate—five grains (.3) of white precipitate, vaseline one ounce (32.)—is the best local dressing.

ANTIMONIUM CRUDUM is the principal internal remedy.

Aconite may be called for in oft repeated doses, if there is much febrile disturbance.

Euphorbium is indicated when there is an irritable skin, with swelling of the face and pea-sized yellow vesicles.

KALI BICH. stands next to Antimonium crud.

Tartar emet., is the remedy when the disease is exceedingly pustular.

THUJA.—After vaccination.

Silicea and Kali nitricum are at times indicated.

INTERTRIGO.

Definition.—Intertrigo is a hyperæmic affection caused by the prolonged contact of two cutaneous surfaces, characterized by heat, redness and an abraded surface with maceration of the epidermis.

Synonyms.—Dermatitis traumatica. Erythema intertrigo. Eczema intertrigo.

Symptomatology.—It is chiefly met with in fat persons and in infants. It may occur whenever the skin hangs in folds, and is therefore more commonly seen about the nates, groin and axillæ, and in the folds of the neck and beneath the mammæ.

Treatment.—The local treatment consists in washing with cold water and castile soap, and after drying with a soft towel, in dusting the parts with lycopodium dust, or oxide of zinc and rice powder equal parts. Attrition of the surfaces should be guarded against.

The principal internal remedies are:

Borax.—Slight injuries ulcerate. Hot urine in infants. Red, papulous itching eruption.

CALCAREA CARB.—Intertrigo in fat, scrofulous children during dentition. Sour vomiting. Hard, distended abdomen.

CHAMOMILLA.—In infants aggravated by every cold change of weather. Child is cross and fretful.

Graphites.—Intertrigo between the thighs with

discharge of glutinous fluid. Itching of the genitals. Aversion to animal food. Slight injuries ulcerate.

Hydrastis.—Irritation maddening, with intense burning heat. Constipation with hæmorrhoids.

Mercurius.—Rawness with great soreness, worse at night. Soreness between the thighs and genitals. Swelling and inflammation of the glands. Superficial, wide-spread ulceration.

Petroleum.—Intertrigo behind the ears. Tips of fingers rough, cracked and fissured. Itching, soreness and moisture of the genitals. Painful sensitiveness of the skin.

Psoricum.—Intolerable itching in the evening and at night. Offensive perspiration at the anus and perineum.

Arsenicum sulphide, Nux juglans and Lycopodium may be compared in chronic and obstinate cases.

ITCH.

Definition.—See Scabies.

KELOID.

Definition.—Keloid is an affection of the skin, characterized by the development of one or more flattish smooth-surfaced tumors, usually upon the site of cicatrices.

Synonyms.—Cheloid. Kelis.

Symptomatology.—The form of the tumor is very variable, and somewhat peculiar, in that it is usually made up of a central portion or body, having numerous prolongations or claws. It may vary in size from a five-cent piece, to several centimeters in diameter. Its usual seat is the sternum and mammæ, though it may appear on other parts. It is a disease mainly of adult life, and is seen oftenest in colored people.

The tumors are slightly painful on pressure, but do not tend toward ulceration. Spontaneous evolution occasionally takes place.

Treatment.—Excision is not attended by good results, as the tumor is prone to return in the scar. Galvanism by means of surface applications, does more than anything else in the way of local treatment.

Fluoric acid, is the principal internal remedy, and the next is *Graphites.*

Nitric acid and Sabina, are occasionally indicated.

LENTIGO.

Definition.—Lentigo is a skin discoloration due to deposit of pigment in the rete mucosum, and is characterized by round yellowish split-pea sized spots.

Synonym.—Freckles.

Symptomatology.—It appears for the most part on the cheeks and back of the hands, and is seen more in light complexioned, and especially red haired people.

Treatment.—The best local application is the ointment of the oleate of copper, prepared by dissolving one drachm (4.) of the salt of oleate of copper in sufficient oleo-palmitic acid to make a soft ointment. It may be applied every night on retiring. Night and morning applications of a mercuric bichloride lotion, two grains (.13) to the ounce (32.), are frequently of service.

The internal remedies are:

Ferrum mag.—Spots resembling summer freckles on back of hands and fingers.

KALI CARB.—Freckles on the face.

Lycopodium.—Freckles on the left side of the face and across the nose.

Nitric acid.—Freckles on the chest. Dark freckles.

Petroleum.—Freckles on the arms.

Phosphorus.—Freckles on the lower limbs.

SEPIA.—Freckles on the cheeks.

SULPHUR.—Freckles on the nose.

LEPROSY.

Definition.—Leprosy is a constitutional disease, occurring endemically in some countries, and characterized by the occurrence of cellular deposits in the skin and other tissues, producing changes which usually result in the destruction of the parts, with anæsthesia and great deformity.

Synonyms.—Leontiasis. Lepra. Elephantiasis græcorum.

Symptomatology.—This is supposed to be the leprosy alluded to in the Bible, and was the leprosy of Europe in the middle ages.

It occurs principally in warm climates and is common along the shores of the Mediterranean, and in India, Japan and China, in the Sandwich Islands, Brazil and the West Indies.

In the United States it has been seen among the Chinese in California, and in a Norwegian community in Minnesota, and from statistics is certainly on the increase. Leprosy exhibits several different phases, and according to the predominance of certain lesions or symptoms, may be divided into three sets, viz: The *tubercular* the *macular* and the *anœsthetic*.

A prodromal stage of gradual decline in health, running for weeks, months, or even years, generally precedes the more decided and characteristic features. Faint brownish patches of the size of a nickel or larger, often mistaken for syphilitic maculation, show themselves. Oftentimes an eruption of bullæ followed by slight scars and pigmentation is one of the first symptoms.

The macules as they increase in size peripherally, retain their brownish color at the edges, but gradually fade into dirty gray color in the centre. When first formed the patches are markedly hyperæsthetic, while later they may become completely anæsthetic. They may appear on any part of the body, but are commonly seen on the trunk, and extensor surfaces of the extremities.

In connection with the maculæ or independently, dull brownish-red tubercles, roundish in form, and varying in size from a pea to a large plum, may make their appearance. These form in greatest numbers on the face, and by obliterating the natural lines, give rise to a peculiar *leonine* expression. After a time tubercles may appear upon the mucous membrane of the buccal cavity, nares and larynx. Ulceration takes place sooner or later, from the breaking down and softening of the tubercles. The hair and nails fall out.

The fingers and toes become bent and crooked, caries set in, and one by one the phalanges disintegrate or finally drop off. The average duration of leprosy is about fifteen years.

Diagnosis.—Well marked leprosy can hardly be mistaken for any other disease.

In the early stage when the macules are small and pinkish, it may be mistaken for a papulo-macular syphilide. Later, when the tubercles are arranged in aggregated patches, it closely resembles lupus.

The spots of leprosy are, however, larger, more infiltrated and tender, smoother and change to a darker color than in syphilis.

The nodules of leprosy are firmer, tender and more oily than are the tubercles of lupus.

Prognosis.—The prognosis is unfavorable.

Treatment.—As tending to prevent the spread of leprosy, the sequestration of those attacked in infected districts should be enjoined. A generous diet with plenty of fresh air and out door exercise is of vital importance.

Cod liver oil, or what is better, Chaulmoogra oil may be taken in such quantities and as often as the stomach will permit.

Locally, warm baths with Gurjun oil are highly recommended.

The principal internal remedies are HYDROCOTYLE, HOANG NAN and *Piper methysticum.*

Others may be indicated as follows:

Arsenicum alb.—Hyperæsthesia followed soon by

anæsthesia. General prostration. Burning like fire in parts of the body. Loss of hair and eyebrows. Livid tubercles on any part of the body.

ARSENICUM IODAT.—Pricking sensation in the skin. Loss of the voice. Enlargement of the glands. Hoarse cough. Falling off of the fingers and toes. Ozæna. Tubercles dirty looking.

Aurum.—Melancholy disposition. Discharge from the nares very offensive. Absorption of the bones of the nose. Has no desire to talk about sickness.

CALOTROPIS GIG.—In tubercular leprosy.

Crotalus.—Swelling of the limbs or body. Spots appearing like gangrene.

Cuprum.—Leprous eruptions. Cramps. Suffocating spells.

GRAPHITES.—Obstruction of the nares. Skin cracks and discharges a sticky fluid. Leprous spots. Coppery annular raised spots on the face, buttocks, legs and feet. Ulcers on the toes.

HYDROCOTYLE.—Well marked cases of tubercular leprosy. Leonine face. Nose flattened and swollen. Lobes of the ears pendulous and swollen. Ulcers in the alæ nasi and corners of the mouth. Ears discharge. Hands and feet swollen so that fingers and toes spread apart. Itching of any part of body. Feeling of lassitude. Yellowish or reddish spots on the trunk and extremities.

Iodum.—Emaciation marked. Swelling of the glands. When mercury has been taken in large quantities. Loss of voice and hoarseness. Voracious appetite.

Kali bich.—Brownish colored spots. Ulcers with an unhealthy look. Blisters on the extremities. Little boils or pustules on any part of body. Thick, tough discharge from nose. Hard plugs in nose. Thick, yellow, putrid discharge from the ears. Ulcers on tongue and on cornea.

Kreosot.—Sores on the nose. Swollen gums. Painful ulcers. Wheals like urticaria. Numbness in different parts of the body.

Lachesis.—Large boils. Bloody serum discharge from the nose, ears and mouth. Obstinate ulcers with black spot in the granulations. Ulcers on the cornea.

Mercurius.—Falling out of the teeth. Absorption of small bones. Swollen gums. Sore tongue. Flat indolent ulcers.

Petroleum.—Tubercles on the face. Unhealthy skin with brown spots. Skin dries and forms deep cracks. Falling out of hair. Ulcers on fingers and tibia. Hyperæsthesia of scalp and ears followed by anæsthesia. Ravenous appetite. Numbness of extremities.

Phosphorus.—In latter stages. Boils. Hair falls out. Spots like blood blisters on the body. Great debility with increase of sexual desire.

Rhus.—Scalp sensitive, cannot bear to have the hair touched. Pulsation in the ears. Loss of smell. Swollen face so that patient is not recognized. Tubercles with sharply defined margins. Bright red skin, violent itching. Hardness and thickening of skin on any part of body.

Secale.—Can hardly talk, the tongue will not respond to the will. Fingers and toes drop off. Falling out of the hair. Eyes look sunken. Cold, dried up looking skin.

Sepia.—Breath offensive. Loss of smell. Red eyes. Falling out of the hair and eyebrows. Brownish spots on face. Skin peels off from hands and feet. Nails look dried up and deformed. Swollen forehead and temples. Face thick and covered with tubercles. Leonine face. Drawing ulcers on fingers and toes.

Silicea.—White spots on face. Shortening of ham strings. Induration of nose with ulceration and discharge.

Woorari.—Obstinate boils that will not heal. Slowly forming and suppurating pimples. Dirty looking skin. Blood oozes through the skin. Tubercles on nose. Stoppage of nose with swelling of parts. Falling out of hair. Swelling of the lobes of ears. Falling out of the teeth. Discharge of matter from the ears. Tonsils inflame and suppurate.

Hura Braziliensis, Guano and Helleborus fœtidus may be compared.

LEUCODERMA.

Definition.—Leucoderma is a cutaneous disease, characterized by localized loss of pigment. Congenital absence of pigment is called *albinism*.

Synonyms.—Cutis variegata. Piebald skin.

Symptomatology.—Leucoderma is a rare affection, and seldom appears before adult life. The general health is as a rule good, though the nervous system may at times be implicated. The face, hands and genitals are usually the parts first invaded. The patches are either round or oval, and are of a milk white color. They may either increase in size or remain stationary, and seldom if ever, regain their normal color.

Diagnosis.—Leucoderma is to be distinguished from leprosy, chloasma, tinea versicolor and morphœa.

Treatment.—Of the treatment nothing encouraging can be said. Locally, the pigmentation around the patch may be lessened by the use of strong acetic acid. Galvanism may prove serviceable. Internally the SULPHIDE OF ARSENICUM will be oftenest used with benefit. Natrum, Nitric acid, Sumbul and the Phosphide of Zinc may be studied.

LICHEN PLANUS.

Definition.—Lichen planus is a chronic disease characterized by the appearance of dull-red, flat-topped, angular-based pin-head sized glazed papules, running a distinctly papular course, and attended by more or less pruritus.

Symptomatology.—It is a rare disease in this country, and is usually associated with a debilitated state of the system, depending upon a faulty nutrition. The eruption generally makes its appearance in the form of solid, millet-seed sized papules, that in the early stages have a shiny aspect, but later on are covered with thin micaceous scales. They start abruptly from the skin, are irregular shaped, flattened on the top and frequently present in the center an umbilicated depression, which is the opening of the hair follicle. They are usually discrete, but may be aggregated in patches, and as a rule develop slowly and occur symmetrically. Melasmic stains frequently, and little pits occasionally remain after the disappearance of the papules.

The disease may occur at any time of life, attacks women more than men, and selects as seats the front of the forearms and wrists, the thighs, abdomen, and the legs below the knees. It arises primarily as a disturbance of the trophic nerves of the hair papilla, with resulting hyperæmia and formation of new tissue.

Diagnosis.—Lichen planus is to be distinguished from papular eczema and papular syphilide.

Prognosis.—The prognosis is usually favorable, except in the diffuse form of the disease, the *lichen ruber* of Hebra, which is commonly associated with marasmus, and may terminate fatally.

Treatment.—The patient should be liberally fed and well hygiened. Local treatment may be resorted to mainly to allay the annoying itching.

ANTIMONIUM CRUD. is the principal internal remedy.

Others are indicated as follows:

Agaricus musc.—Eruption of small pimples with red areolæ and violent itching. Sensation in various parts as if ice cold needles were piercing the skin. In light complexioned persons and drunkards.

ARSENICUM ALB.—In chronic cases. Burning itching, painful after scratching. Great weakness and prostration. Oppression of breathing.

Chinium ars.—In the diffused form with threatening marasmus. Chronic intestinal derangements.

Iodine.—Small dry, red pimples on the arms, chest and back, with jerking sensation while appearing. Rough, dry skin. Emaciation. Ravenous hunger.

KALI BICH.—Papular eruptions on the forearms. Rheumatic pains in the limbs. In fat light complexioned individuals.

LEDUM.—Eruption of pimples on the forehead as in brandy drinkers. Eruption of small pimples like red millet seeds over the body. Excessive itching on the backs of both feet, worse after scratching, and by warmth of bed. Relieved after scratching the feet sore.

NUX JUGLANS.—Red pimples on face, neck, shoulders and back. Little tubercles with hard scurf on the instep.

Potassium iodide.—Lichen on the face and shoulders. Sensitive swelling of the thyroid gland. Great general debility.

Sarsaparilla.—Red dry pimples. Burning itching with chilliness.

Staphysagria.—Itching pimply eruption over the face and behind the ears, with rough skin. Burning of the eruption after scratching.

Sulphur iodide.—Red pimples on the nose, chin and arms, with itching. In chronic cases.

LICHEN SIMPLEX.

Definition.—Lichen simplex is a disease characterized by round solid millet seed sized flesh colored or reddish papules, running a distinctly papular course, and accompanied by marked itching.

Symptomatology.—It is one of the rarer diseases, and appears for the most part in summer time. At the dispensary it constitutes about three per cent. of all skin affections. The papules are usually seen on the outer aspects of the forearm, the neck and the thighs. They last a week or more, and disappear by resorption. Frequently the disease attacks the backs of the hands, which may secondarily become inflamed, and give out a discharge (L. agrius.)

When the papules are seated at the hair follicles, it has been termed (L. pilaris.)

Treatment.—The lotions recommended in eczema to allay the itching may be used in this disease. Bran baths may also be of service.

The indicated internal remedy will generally be one of the following:

Alumina.—Red pimples on the face. Pimples on the neck and back. Intolerable itching of the whole body, especially when becoming heated in bed.

Ammonium mur.—Pimples on the back of the hands desquamating next day.

Anatherium.—Red pimples with itching and burning. Scarlet skin with burning.

Antimonium crud.—Small red pimples on right shoulder. From digestive derangement.

Arsenicum alb.—In chronic cases with burning itching.

Belladonna.—Papular eruption on the hands like lichen agrius.

Bovista.—Red pimples on the foot.

Bryonia.—Pimples on the abdomen and hips.

Castanea vesca.—Several small pimples on the right thigh, back of the left ear, and on the left upper lip.

Caladium.—Pimples on the mons veneris. Soreness of pimples to the touch.

Kreasotum.—Forehead covered with pimples the size of millet seeds.

Ledum.—Small pimples like red millet seeds over the whole body. In brandy drinkers.

Mercurius.—Pimples on the labia. Voluptuous itching. Itching changes to burning by scratching.

Nabulus serpent.—Pimples on the face about the nose, upper lip and chest with itching.

Natrum carb.—Pimples on the face and lips. White pimples on the nose.

Nux juglans.—Red pimples on the face and neck. Pricking itching.

Plantago maj.—Hard white flattened isolated papules on the inside of the thigh. Some papules have a red point in the centre.

Phytolacca.—Pimples with itching on the left leg. Worse first part of the night.

Rumex crisp.—Red pimples on calves of the legs, with itching worse immediately after undressing.

Sepia.—Pimples close together on the face. Pimples on the legs, and in the bends of the joints.

SULPHUR.—Pimples on inner parts of the thighs. In simple cases.

Sulphur iodide.—Red pimples on the nose, chin and arms.

Tilia.—Eruption of small red, rather deeply seated pimples, with violent itching and burning like fire after scratching.

LUPUS ERYTHEMATOSUS.

Definition.—Lupus erythematosus has been defined as characterized by one or more usually roundish or oval, variably sized reddish patches, covered with fine thin whitish or grayish fatty adherent scales.

Synonyms.—Erythematous scrofulide. Lupus sebaceus. Seborrhœa congestiva.

Symptomatology.—The disease appears at the outset as pin-head sized, pale red spots or patches, situated for the most part upon the cheeks and nose. Their centres, occasionally marked by comedo-points of a greenish hue, usually correspond to the orifices of the hair follicles, which are widely distended and patulous. They tend to coalesce and form patches, and are covered with firmly adherent fatty scales. These patches extend gradually by their peripheries, at times healing in the centre, where the skin presents a whitish sunken, as if thinned, appearance. Lupus erythematosus is one of the rarer skin affections, and usually tends to become chronic. It seldom occurs before the twentieth year of life, attacks females more than males and more especially those who are subject to disorders of the sebaceous glands. It is generally confined to the face, and when fully developed presents a peculiar configuration that has been likened to a bat with outspread wings. The body of the bat corresponding to the nose and the wings to the cheeks.

Lupus erythematosus is usually regarded as a chronic inflammation of the skin, leading to degeneration and atrophy.

Diagnosis.—From lupus vulgaris, it is distinguished by the fact that the tubercles and ulcers of the former are never seen in the latter. The sebaceous glands are disordered in lupus erythematosus, not in lupus vulgaris. Lupus vulgaris appears during childhood ; lupus erythematosus is a disease of adult life.

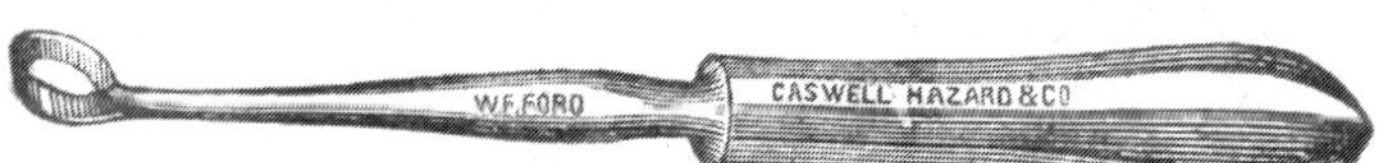

FIG. 9. DERMAL CURETTE.

Prognosis.—The prognosis should be guarded, as relapses are liable to occur.

Treatment.—The diet should be of the best quality and generous. Fresh air and frequent bathing are valuable adjuvants. Saponaria bark or sulphur baths are often of service.

In severe and obstinate cases resort may be had to the curette or scoop (Fig. 9).

IODINE is the principal internal remedy. Guaraca, Hydrocotyle, Cistus, Sepia, and Apis may be compared.

LUPUS VULGARIS.

Definition.—Lupus vulgaris is a disease of the skin characterized by variously shaped, pea-sized or larger, yellowish or reddish elevations, which are soft and pulpy and usually terminate in ulceration and cicatrization.

Synonyms.—Tubercular scrofulide. Lupus exedens. Noli me tangere. Lupus tuberculosus.

Symptomatology.—It usually begins in the form of yellowish or reddish solid points, at first disseminated but later tending to aggregate in patches. They are firm and painless, and gradually enlarge to form papules and tubercles that vary in size from a pin's head to a split pea, and are covered with a thin layer of adherent epidermis. (L. tuberculosus). Later the process may terminate either by insensible absorption of the lupus tissue, commencing with its degeneration and followed, without ulceration, by thinning of the textures with marked scaliness (L. exfoliativus); or terminating in a free breaking down of the neoplasm with destruction of the infiltrated structure and resulting ulceration followed by atrophic cicatrices, (L. exedens).

Lupus vulgaris, is one of the most chronic and obstinate of skin affections. It occurs mostly about the age of puberty, selects scrofulous subjects, and attacks by preference, the face and extremities. The cartilages, fibrous tissues and mucous membrane are its favorite seats.

It is a rare disease in this country, though common in Europe.

Diagnosis.—It may at times be mistaken for syphilis. The hard rapidly developed tubercles of syphilis, however, differ greatly from the soft slow growing "apple jelly" ones of lupus. The ulcers of syphilis have sharply defined borders, and discharge a copious offensive secretion; those of lupus are illy defined, and have a slight and inoffensive discharge. The crusts of syphilis are bulky, and of a greenish color; those of lupus are scanty and of a brownish-red color. The cicatrices of syphilis are soft and whitish; those of lupus are shrunken and yellowish.

Lupus may also be confounded with epithelioma. But if it is remembered that the hard everted edges of the latter are never seen in the former, and that the former is a disease of childhood and youth, while the latter is confined mostly to adult life, the mistake will rarely be made.

Prognosis.—The prognosis is usually good when the lesion is small, but becomes less favorable as it increases in size. Occasionally the disease disappears spontaneously.

Treatment.—An abundant supply of fresh air and outdoor exercise, along with a nutritious diet, is of the utmost importance in the treatment of this disease.

In the earlier stages the red iodide of mercury ointment—red iodide of mercury two drachms (8.) vaseline two drachms (8.)—will be found serviceable as a superficial destructive.

Later the papules or tubercles may be bored with an irido-platinum needle (Fig. 10) dipped two or three times in Squibb's fused nitrate and allowed to cool. Smaller and less painful punctures can be made with these needles than with any other appliances.

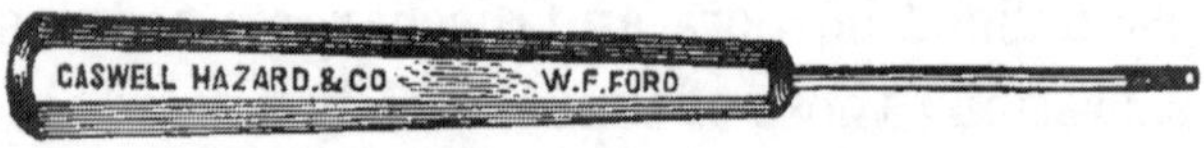

FIG. 10. IRIDO-PLATINUM NEEDLE.

The arsenical mucilage alluded to in the treatment of epithelioma is also useful. At the Dispensary a ten per cent. ointment of pyrogallic acid has been used with very satisfactory results.

In severe cases erasion with the curette or scoop (Fig. 9) and multiple scarification are of great service.

ARSENICUM ALB. and HYDROCOTYLE, are the main internal remedies.

Others may be indicated as follows:

Aurum mur.—When starting from the nasal mucous membrane. Discharge from the nares very offensive. Absorption of the bones of the nose. Melancholy disposition.

Calcium sulphide.—Lupus on the elbows. Ulcers with burning or stinging edges. Nodosities on the head sore to the touch. Swelling of the upper lip.

CISTUS.—Lupus on the face. Worse from cold air.

GRAPHITES.—Lupus on the nose. Obstruction of the nares. Dry, cracked skin. Every injury tends to ulceration.

Guaraca trich.—Lupus of an ochre-red color. Yellow spots on the temples.

Hydrastis.—Ulcers on the legs. Exfoliation of the skin. Purulent discharge from the nostrils. Faint, sinking feeling at the stomach.

Kali bich.—Ulcers painful to the touch. Worse in cold weather. Ulceration of the nasal septum. Loss of appetite. All the secretions are tenacious and stringy.

Lycopodium.—In recent cases. Hunger with constant feeling of satiety. Arms and fingers go to sleep easily. Purulent discharge from the ears. Weakness of memory. Melancholia.

Nitric acid.—Lupus on the lobules of the ears. Offensive purulent discharge from the ears. Dry, scaly skin. Affections of the bones and glands. In dark complexioned individuals.

Staphysagria.—Ulcers on the alæ of the nose. Weary pains in the limbs as if bruised. Teeth turn black and decay. In scrofulous subjects.

MILIARIA.

Definition.—Miliaria is a disease of the skin due to a disordered action of the sweat glands, characterized by the formation of numerous pin-head sized reddened papules or vesico-papules, attended with heat and tingling.

Symptomatology.—The usual seat of the eruption is the trunk, but it may also appear upon the face, neck and arms. It is extremely fitful in its character, frequently appearing and disappearing many times in twenty-four hours.

The disease occurs more during summer time, and when the weather changes suddenly to hot. Superflous clothing is a quite frequent cause. Miliaria is apt to relapse in successive years.

Treatment.—A weak carbolated bran bath, followed by dusting with either the nitrate of bismuth and starch, or lycopodium powder is the best local treatment.

Internally, BRYONIA is the principal remedy. *Arsenicum alb.*, Centaurea, Hura Braziliensis, Ledum and Raphanus may be studied.

MILIUM.

Definition.—Milium is a disorder of the sebaceous glands, characterized by the formation of white, roundish sebaceous points beneath the epidermis.

Synonyms.—Grutum. Acne punctata albida. Strophulus albidus.

Symptomatology.—The white papules look like grains of sand. They occur mostly on the forehead and eyelids, and are more common in women than in men. They vary in size from a millet seed to a split pea, and are generally painless.

The "skin-stones" or cutaneous calculi occasionally met with are generally milia which have undergone calcareous degeneration.

Treatment.—The local treatment consists in opening each milium with an ordinary lancet, and removing the more or less hardened contents. To facilitate removal the milium needle (Fig. 11) may be used.

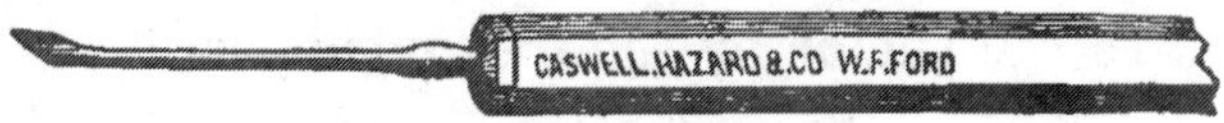

FIG. 11. MILIUM NEEDLE.

To prevent the return of the milia the skin may be washed in saponaria bark water, and afterwards gently rubbed.

The CALCIUM IODIDE is the most important internal remedy, and the next, STAPHYSAGRIA. Tabacum may be thought of.

MITE-DISEASE.

Symptomatology.—Mite disease is found in the south-western states, especially along the Mississippi river, and is due to the *leptus irritans*, or irritating harvest-mite or "jigger."

It occurs usually in summer and autumn, along the banks of rivers and in swampy places.

The mite burrows in the skin, generally of the ankles and legs, and causes considerable irritation, resulting in the formation of papules, vesicles and pustules.

Treatment.—Mild parasiticides, of which *sulphur ointment* is the type, will readily remove the trouble.

Ledum is the principal internal remedy.

MOLLUSCUM SEBACEUM.

Definition.—Molluscum sebaceum is a disease of the sebaceous glands, characterized by roundish pea-sized tumors, umbilicated in the centre and of a pinkish-white color.

Synonyms.—Molluscum contagiosum. Acne molluscum.

Symptomatology.—The umbilicated appearance is given to the tumor by the distended gland duct, from which a white, cheesy matter may be squeezed.

At times the disease appears to be semi-epidemic, but it has not as yet been clearly demonstrated to be contagious.

It is mainly a disease of children, and attacks more especially the face, though it may appear on other parts.

Treatment.—In the early stages touching the parts once or twice a day with the acid nitrate of mercury is often of decided benefit. If the tumors are large, they may be removed by the knife or curved scissors.

SILICEA as an internal remedy ranks first, and *Teucrium* next. Bryonia, Bromine, *Calc. ars.*, Lycopodium, Natrum mur. and Potassium iodide complete the list.

MORPHŒA.

Definition.—Morphœa is a rare disease, characterized by roundish dirty alabaster looking, firm inelastic patches circumscribed by lilac-tinted borders, and varying in diameter from one to three inches.

Synonym.—Addison's keloid.

Symptomatology.—It usually commences as a delicate purple-colored spot, in the centre of which a pale area shows itself. This central spot becomes more and more decided as it grows, and finally assumes the appearance of a piece of white wax, depressed and surrounded by a lilac-tinted ring.

At times the patches become the seats of irregular deposits of pigment, and as the disease progresses atrophic changes are apt to take place in the affected parts.

Morphœa occurs more in woman than in men, and selects the course of the left supra-orbital nerve as its most frequent seat. The corium appears bound down to the subcutaneous tissue, and the skin is leather-like.

It runs an extremely slow course, and occasionally terminates in spontaneous recovery.

Etiology.—It is supposed to be of neurotic origin.

Diagnosis.—It may be mistaken for scleroderma, leprosy, or leucoderma. It never has the sclerodermic hardness of scleroderma. Leprosy never has the waxy patches of morphœa. Leucoderma is simply a pigmentary disease, and as such does not present the textural changes of morphœa.

Treatment.—The patient should be well fed, and have a daily allowance of either cod liver or chaulmoogra oil. Locally, the constant galvanic current, with daily phosphorated oil inunctions is beneficial.

PHOSPHORUS is the principal internal remedy.

NÆVUS.

Definition.—Nævus is a congenital formation, seated in the skin and subcutaneous tissue, and may be either pigmentary or vascular.

Synonyms.—Claret stain. Port-wine stain. Mother's mark. Birth mark. Pigmentary mole.

Symptomatology.—*Pigmentary nœvi* are dark-colored, slightly elevated, sharply defined spots, varying in size from a pin's head to a fifty-cent piece. When covered with hair they are called "mouse marks" (*nævus pilosus.*)

Vascular nævi are the commoner of the two, and may be either *arterial* (fire-marks) or *venous*. They are of a reddish or purplish color, and may be large or small. They are met with on all parts of the body, have a variable course, and may elect to increase in size, remain stationary, or disappear.

A vascular nævus consists of an aggregation of dilated bloodvessels, the walls of which are frequently thickened, and the plexuses arranged irregularly.

Treatment.—The pigmentary nævi may be removed by the application of sodium ethylate, prepared by adding the metal sodium to absolute alcohol. Sodium ethylate is best applied by means of a glass rod.

The vascular nævi are best treated by either electrolysis or the subcutaneous ligature.

When treated by electrolysis one or several platinum needles connected with the negative pole of an ordinary zinc and carbon battery of six or twelve cells are introduced into the nævus, the positive pole being placed above. After from ten to thirty seconds the needles are removed and the growth will present a bluish-white appearance. With proper care neither sloughing nor suppuration will occur.

In superficial circumscribed nævi, multiple puncture with fine needles dipped in a twenty-five or fifty per cent. solution of chromic acid has been used with success.

CARBO VEG. is the principal internal remedy for the pigmentary nævus, and THUJA for the vascular. Calcarea carb., and Condurango may be compared.

NETTLE-RASH.

Definition.—See Urticaria.

ONYCHAUXIS.

Definition.—Onychauxis manifests itself by simple increase in the normal growth of the nail.

Treatment.—GRAPHITES is the remedy.

ONYCHIA.

Definition.—Onychia is an inflammation of the matrix of the nail.

Symptomatology.—It may occur in the course of such diseases as eczema, psoriasis and syphilis, or may be due to local injury.

Treatment.—For simple onychia FLUORIC ACID is the internal remedy. When occurring from a bruise or other injury, ARNICA both internally and externally, proves serviceable.

ONYCHOGRYPHOSIS.

Definition.—Onychogryphosis is characterized by a twisted bent condition of the nails, which are thickened and of a yellowish or brownish color. It affects mostly the nails of the toes and fingers, and generally attacks old people.

Treatment.—*Graphites* and *Silicea* are the main remedies.

ONYCHO-MYCOSIS.

Definition.—Onycho-mycosis is a disease generally confined to one nail, and is due to the ravages of one of the vegetable parasites.

See Tinea tricophytina.

PARONYCHIA.

Definition.—Paronychia is an inflammation situated around and beneath the nail, terminating in suppuration.

Synonym.—Run-around.

Symptomatology.—It attacks mostly the thumb and fingers, and makes its appearance as a dusky-red, extremely painful border, either completely or partially surrounding the nail. In a few days the pain becomes throbbing in character and pus forms, attended at times by more or less constitutional disturbance.

A form of this affection is sometimes caused by ingrowing of the nail, and more especially the nail of the big toe.

Diagnosis.—Paronychia differs from whitlow or felon, in that the latter involves all or nearly all the structures of the fingers, and appears for the most part on the *palmar* surfaces.

Treatment.—Locally, the pith of the common *bulrush* has been used with good results.

NATRUM SULPH., is the principal internal remedy. In slight cases *Graphites* often proves beneficial, and when suppuration is tardy, Calcium sulphide renders excellent service. Rana bufo is useful when there are red streaks up the arm.

PEMPHIGUS.

Definition.—Pemphigus is a cutaneous disease, characterized by the appearance of bullæ, usually in groups of three or four, and varying in size from a pea to a hickory nut.

Synonym.—Pompholyx.

Symptomatology.—The disease is almost always chronic and may exist in either of two forms, namely: *P. foliaceus* and *P. vulgaris.*

Pemphigus vulgaris is most common upon the limbs and more especially about the ankles. Occasionally it appears on the mucous membrane and other parts of the body.

The blisters or bullæ are rounded or oval, and rise abruptly from the skin sometimes to the height of a centimeter or more, and may be attended by slight itching. Their contents are at first colorless, but later they become cloudy or milky. They usually appear in *successive crops*, each bulla running its course in from four to five days.

Acute pemphigus is rarely met with, excepting in children. It runs its course in from three to six weeks, and relapses are prone to occur.

Pemphigus foliaceus attacks the body generally, and is often a fatal though rare form of disease.

It usually commences by the appearance of a single *flaccid* bulla on the sternum, and from there spreads over the whole surface.

The bullæ differ from those of pemphigus vulgaris, in that they do not become tense, but remain flaccid and dry up to form yellowish parchment-like flakes, which vary in size from one-third of an inch to two inches.

Treatment.—The patient should be placed on a full animal diet, with plenty of fresh air and exercise.

Such means should be used as may tend to bring the health up to its accustomed standard.

Locally, bran, starch or gelatine baths are of decided benefit. The continuous bath, as recommended by Hebra, may be resorted to in some cases.

RHUS TOX., is the principal internal remedy for *acute pemphigus vulgaris*, and ARSENICUM ALB., for the *chronic* form.

THUJA is oftenest indicated in the *foliaceus* variety.

Others may be indicated as follows:

Ammonium mur.—Blisters the size of peas on the right shoulder with itching. Burning at small spots on the chest. Chilliness especially when walking. Fat body but thin legs.

Belladonna.—Painful, watery vesicles on the palm of the hand sensitive to the touch. Chill in the evening, mostly on the arms, with heat in the head.

CAUSTICUM.—Large painful blisters on the left side of the chest and neck, which become flattened. Anguish in the chest with fever. Involuntary urination when sneezing or blowing the nose.

Gummi gutti.—May be used when other remedies fail.

PHOSPHORIC ACID.—Deep hard bullæ on the ball of the thumb. Blisters on the balls of the toes. Great drowsiness and apathy. In debilitated individuals. After sexual excesses.

Phosphorus.—Painful hard blisters, full to bursting. Chilliness every evening with shivering. Arms and hands become numb. Regurgitation of food. Small wounds bleed much.

RANUNCULUS BULB.—Blisters on the fingers the size of a hazel nut, followed after healed by small deep transparent dark-blue elevated blisters the size of ordinary pin-heads.

Raphanus.—Blisters full of water on the breast, without inflammation redness or pain.

Sepia.—Pemphigus on the arms and hands. Heaviness of the limbs. Sensitive to cold air. Arthritic pains in the joints.

PERNIO.

Definition.—Pernio is an inflammation of the skin, occurring as a secondary effect of cold, and appearing for the most part upon the hands and feet.

Synonyms.—Chilblains. Erythema pernio.

Symptomatology.—Occasionally pernio attacks the nose and ears, and may appear on any part of the body. It commences after exposure to cold, by slight vesication attended with tingling, itching, burning sensations. In mild cases it may terminate in a few days with desquamation. In severer cases, remissions and exacerbations are prone to occur and thus prolong the disease for months. The parts are usually left in an irritable state, and are liable to renewed attacks from the slightest causes. Any sudden change of temperature, and especially a combination of cold and moisture, may renew the trouble. In chronic cases the parts become livid or purplish in color, and are more or less swollen and itchy. Ulcers not unfrequently form.

Prognosis.—Pernio when it becomes chronic may last for years, disappearing usually in the summer time,but returning again as winter approaches.

Treatment.—When there is much inflammation a *decoction of marsh mallows*, locally, acts well.

Tamus communis tincture, is recommended as a topical remedy for unbroken chilblains.

Broken chilblains may be dressed with either *oxide of zinc ointment*, or the *glycerole of calendula.*

Resin ointment is adapted to the ulcers that sometimes follow.

The *galvanic* current acts favorably in most cases.

The *tincture of benzoin*, painted on the parts once or twice a day, acts as a preventive.

The remedies likely to prove beneficial are:

Agaricus.—Violent itching, worse at night. Burning in the fingers, lower limbs and toes. Itching, burning and redness of the toes. Muscular twitchings.

Arsenicum alb.—Ulcerated chilblains. Red spots on the feet. Violent tearing pains in edges of ulcers when exposed to cold. Relieved by warm applications.

Badaiga.—Flesh and integuments sore to the touch. Sensitive to cold air.

Belladonna.—Bright red shining swelling, with pulsative pains. Burning in skin when touched. Tingling itching, worse at night.

Cantharis.—Itching and swelling of the fingers. Blisters burning on touch. Burning in the soles of the feet at night in hysteric patients. Tearing and ulcerative pains.

Citrus vulg.—Itching of the swollen hands and arms. General itching which prevents sleep.

Nitric acid.—Itching of the feet. Spreading blisters on the toes. Ulcers with stinging and pricking pains as of splinters. Offensive profuse perspiration on the feet, causing soreness.

Petroleum.—Broken chilblains with tendency to fester. Heel painfully swollen and red with stitches. Tips of fingers rough, cracked and fissured with sticking cutting pain. Unhealthy skin.

Prunus spinosa.—Itching on tips of fingers as if frozen.

Pulsatilla.—Blue-red chilblains with pricking burning pain, worse toward evening. Redness and swelling of joints with stinging pains. Feet feel hot and swollen with tensive burning pains. Wandering pains.

Rhus tox.—Inflamed chilblains with excessive itching. Aching pains in the legs. Worse before storms and from getting wet.

Sulphur.—Thick red chilblains on the fingers which itch severely when warm. Predisposition to chilblains.

Urtica dioica.—Has been used both internally and externally with good results.

Veratrum vir.—Intense painful itching. Chilblains on the nose. Prickling in the fingers and toes. Used internally and locally.

PHTHIRIASIS.

Definition.—Phthiriasis is a contagious affection due to the presence of pediculi.

Synonyms.—Pediculosis. Morbus pedicularis. Lice disease. Crabs.

Symptomatology.—There are three varieties of this disease, each being the outward demonstration of the ravages of distinct species of pediculi.

The *pediculus capitis* or head louse, gives rise to the variety known as *phthiriasis capitis*. It may be found on all parts of the head, but its favorite seat is the occipital region. Numerous ova or "nits" may be deposited along the shafts of the hair. They exist mostly among the children of the poorer classes, but are quite frequently found on women. They cause considerable irritation not by biting, as imagined, but by inserting their suckers or *haustella* into the pores of the skin, and so distending them as to frequently cause drops of blood to follow on their withdrawal. This irritation together with the scratching it induces gives rise to the development of papules, whose apices when scratched off, present the blood tipped appearance so characteristic of phthiriasis.

The *pediculus vestimenti*, or body louse, has its habitat in the clothing, and attacks the body, giving rise to *phthiriasis corporis*. Its ova are deposited and hatched in the clothing. *P. corporis* is mainly a disease of adult years, and is seen mostly in the lower walks of life. The lesions are multiform, due principally to scratching, and have their chief seats on the trunk, hips and thighs.

The *pediculus pubis* or crab louse, usually infests the hair of the pubis, but may wander to other parts. It attacks adults mostly.

The pediculi are air-breathing insects and remain wholly upon the external surface.

Treatment.—The treatment is mainly local, and consists in the destruction of the parasites and their ova. Phthiriasis capitis responds readily to repeated dusting with powdered staphysagria. Cocculus indicus tincture, often proves serviceable. Ordinary petroleum is a most effective application. White precipitate ointment—ten grains (.6) of white precipitate to the ounce (32.) of cosmoline—is useful when "scratch-marks" prove troublesome. The "nits" may be removed by repeated washing with carbolized water.

Phthiriasis corporis is best treated by staphysagria ointment—two drachms (8.) to the ounce (32.)—well rubbed in. The patient's clothing should be thoroughly boiled or baked, so as to ensure the destruction of whatever pediculi may have made it their habitation.

For phthiriasis pubis either cocculus indicus tincture, a mercuric bichloride lotion, or a chloroform application proves an effectual remedy.

Internally, *Oleander* may be given in phthiriasis capitis, and *Mercurius* in the other varieties if desired.

PITYRIASIS.

Definition.—Pityriasis is a cutaneous affection characterized by fine dry bran-like scales, seated on a slightly reddened non-infiltrated surface.

Synonym.—Branny tetter.

Symptomatology.—It affects mostly the scalp, face and upper part of the body, and seldom or never becomes general. If left to itself it is apt to become chronic and last for years. When occurring on the scalp it tends to cause falling of the hair. It is accompanied by slight itching, and may be caused either by heat, cold winds, or local irritants. The disease is seated in the deep layers of the epidermis, and consists in excessive cell proliferation.

Treatment.—Locally an infusion of *saponaria bark* is the best remedy. If the affection is located on the hairy scalp it may be necessary to cut the hair. Glycerole of borax—two drachms (8.) of borax to one ounce (32.) of glycerine—is frequently of service.

ARSENICUM ALB., is the principal internal remedy. Fluoric acid, Colchicum and Kali arsen., are occasionally indicated.

PITYRIASIS RUBRA.

Definition.—See Dermatitis exfoliativa.

PRAIRIE ITCH.

Symptomatology.—Prairie itch is an acute inflammation of the skin, appearing in new districts where it may be for a time endemic. It may be preceded by the premonitory symptoms of malaise, headache, and slight febrile disturbance, or its onset may be first marked by the appearance of erythematous spots, covered with small transparent vesicles, varying in size from a pin's head to a mustard seed and situated for the most part on the neck, shoulders, back and outer surface of the limbs. An intolerable nightly itching accompanies the eruption, creating an almost irresistible desire to scratch the parts. The scratching obliterates the vesicles, and gives rise to scratch marks and to the secretion of an exceedingly acrid irritating fluid, which oftentimes indefinitely prolongs the disease. Large blackish crusts covering suppurating ulcers are an occasional result. Furuncles quite frequently complicate the trouble.

Treatment.—Locally, the diluted lye of wood ashes is the best remedy.

Internally, RUMEX CRISPUS will be oftenest called for. *Rhus tox.*, and Ledum may be studied.

PRURIGO.

Definition.—Prurigo is a disease characterized by the development of small papules, of the same color as the skin, accompanied by intense itching.

Symptomatology.—It commences by the gradual formation of small, sub-epidermic elevations, which have a peculiar shot-like feel, and are frequently perforated by small hairs. These papules are due to chronic inflammatory changes in the papillary layer.

Intense itching or pruritus, with formication is one of the earliest symptoms and generally continues with more or less intensity throughout the entire course of the disease. Hence "scratch marks" are often found complicating the eruption. As the disease progresses the skin becomes thickened and presents a dry, rough, harsh appearance.

Prurigo is mainly an affection of the poorer classes, and occurs mostly on the extensor surfaces of the lower extremities, but is frequently found on the forearms and trunk. It starts as a rule before puberty, becomes aggravated during the winter months, and is apt to continue through life. It is a rare disease in this country. It differs from phthiriasis with which it has been frequently confounded, in that, pediculi which are the cause of the latter are never present in the former.

Diagnosis.—It is to be differentiated from papular eczema and urticaria, and from scabies.

Prognosis.—The prognosis is always doubtful.

Treatment.—A thoroughly nutritious diet should be ordered for the patient. Locally, either tar or sulphur baths are the most serviceable. To allay the itching a carbolic acid, dioscorea, or mezereum lotion may be used.

SULPHUR is the principal remedy for recent attacks, and ARSENICUM IODIDE for the more chronic forms. Ambra, Arsenicum sulphide, Carbolic acid, Dioscorea, Dolichos pruriens, Mercurius, Nitric acid and Oleander may be studied.

PRURITUS.

Definition.—Pruritus, or *simple itching* without any eruption can hardly be called a disease. It is merely a perverted sensation, and is a common accompaniment of a variety of cutaneous affections. When occurring to all appearances independently—as far as any eruption is concerned—it is even then simply symptomatic of some nerve disturbance, indicative of the circulation of bile or some other foreign material in the blood, or else dependent on local excitants.

PSORIASIS.

Definition.—Psoriasis is a constitutional, non-contagious disease of the skin, characterized by reddish thickened patches covered with whitish or yellowish-white mother-of-pearl colored scales.

Synonyms.—Lepra vulgaris. Alphos. Dry or scaly tetter.

Symptomatology.—The patches vary both in size and form. They usually commence as small reddish spots, hardly raised above the skin and covered with whitish scales. As a rule they develop rapidly, so that in a few days they may be as large as a nickel and present the appearance of drops of mortar. Generally the patches tend to run together as they increase in size, and lose the circular outline that at first characterized them. Occasionally the centers of the patches clear up, giving to the disease the appearance of rings. Frequently two rings come in contact with each other at the edges, thus forming the figure 8. At times the circles are incomplete, and as a consequence many lines are formed. Some writers err in speaking of these different stages, as distinct varieties of disease, and so allude to psoriasis punctata, psoriasis nummularis, psoriasis gyrata, etc. Such, however, can not be held to be distinct varieties of cutaneous trouble, but are simply stages of one and the same affection.

The scales of psoriasis are peculiar and characteristic. They are imbricated, of a silvery white color, and situated on a red and inflamed base. The presence of air in the scales is the supposed cause of their white appearance. The favorite seats of the disease are the tips of the elbows, the fronts of the knees and the head. It may, however, appear on any part of the cutaneous surface, and is apt to be symmetrical. It is never seen on the mucous membranes or the red margins of the lips, and is but rarely observed on the palms and soles. In gouty individuals the scales are thin, often scanty, attended with marked itching, and seated on a very red and congested base. In strumous subjects, however, the scales are thick, oftentimes heaped up, attended with but slight itching, and seated on a less congested base.

The involution of the disease is characterized by the diminished elevation of the patch, and the fading of the eruption, which leaves neither staining nor cicatrization.

Etiology.—The etiology of psoriasis is still obscure. By some it is claimed to be of malarial and by others of traumatic origin. The disease is neither contagious nor hereditary. It occurs alike in both sexes, and very rarely appears before puberty. It prevails more in winter than in summer.

Next to eczema it is one of the commonest cutaneous diseases of this country. My experience at the dispensary, ranks it the fourth in order of frequency.

Lang claims to have discovered fungus elements in

psoriasis, which he considers the cause of the disease.

Morbid anatomy.—It forms principally in the upper layers of the corium and on the apices of the papillæ, and is due to a perversion of the cell life of the rete. The scales are made up of masses of cells from the stratum lucidum.

Diagnosis.—The diagnosis of psoriasis is generally easy. It may at times be mistaken for eczema, tinea tricophytina, lichen planus, lupus erythematosus, pityriasis, ichthyosis, and the squamous syphilide. Sufficiently characteristic, however, are the silvery white heaped-up scales, seated on an inflamed cutis which inclines to bleed in pin-point drops on their removal, and the selection of the elbows, knees and head as sites.

Treatment.—The diet in psoriasis should be a generous one, and in it meat ought always to play an important part. Cod liver oil is generally needed.

The local treatment consists in first removing the scales by means of saponaria or bran baths. Inunctions with cod liver oil or chaulmoogra oil may then be resorted to, and especially so, if, as occasionally happens, there is considerable attendant inflammation. In more obstinate cases unless the skin is very irritable the oil of white birch may be used in the form of an ointment, one drachm (4.) to the ounce (32.) of vaseline. Marked success has followed the use of chrysarobin or chrysophanic acid in the form of a cerate, not too strong. One great objection to its use, especially upon uncovered parts, is the mahogany-colored staining that attends it. It may be prepared in strengths varying from ten grains (.66) to one drachm (4.) to the ounce (32.) of vaseline. A fifteen per cent ointment of beta naphthol is recommended by Kaposi, especially in the treatment of psoriatic patches upon the face and scalp.

It is best to commence the internal treatment with SULPHUR. Afterwards one of the following remedies may be given:

Ammonium carb.—White pea-sized spots upon the cheek, which continually exfoliate. Skin very sensitive to cold. Aversion to being washed. Nose bleed when washing the face in the morning. In weak nervous individuals.

ARSENICUM ALB.—Skin dry and scaly. Great restlessness with weakness and prostration. Burning itching. Oppression of breathing. Aggravated by eating fruit, ice cream, etc.

ARSENICUM IODIDE.—Dry scaly burning itching eruption on various parts. Persistent itching on the back. In obstinate cases.

Calcarea carb.—Scurfy spots on the leg. Burning and itching. Skin cracks. Profuse sweat from the slightest exertion. Large abdomen. Blue eyes, blonde hair, fair skin.

Fluoric acid.—Roughness on the forehead like a rough line with its convexity upwards. Reddish spots above the eyebrows. Desquamation on the eyebrows. Nails brittle, edges bent in.

Hydrocotyle.—Circular spots with slightly raised scaly edges.

Iris versicolor.—Irregular psoriatic patches on the knees and elbows, covered with shining scales. Skin fissured and irritable. Gastric and bilious derangements.

Manganum.—In inveterate cases.

MERCURIUS.—Psoriasis of the hands. Psoriasis in spots all over the body. Scaling off and exfoliation of the finger nails. The scalp is painful to the touch. Easy perspiration without relief. In recent cases.

Mezereum.—Scurf-like scales on the back, chest, scalp and thighs. Roughness and scaling here and there. Pruritus increased by scratching or when undressing.

Muriatic acid.—Psoriasis of the hands. Great sensitiveness to damp weather.

NATRUM ARS.—Thin whitish scales, which when removed leave the skin slightly reddened.

Petroleum.—Skin of the hands cracked and rough. Unhealthy skin. Aversion to the open air. Extreme sensitiveness to slight touch. Falling off of the hair.

PHOSPHORUS.—Psoriasis of the arms and hands, and on the knees and elbows. Arms and hands become numb. Coldness of the kees at night in bed. Falling out of the hair in large bunches. Dry cough with soreness in the chest.

Phytolacca.—Surface of the skin shrunken and of a leaden color. Squamous eruption. Rheumatic pains in the extremities.

Selenium.—Dry scaly eruption on the palms of the hands, with slight itching.

Sepia.—Psoriasis on the face. Red roughness of the skin. Falling off of the hair. During pregnancy and nursing. Dark complexioned individuals.

Silicea.—Elevated scurfy spots near the coccyx. Small white scales on the face and neck. White spots on the cheeks. Sensation of numbness in the extremities. Brittleness of the nails. In scrofulous, large bellied children. Imperfect assimilation.

Teucrium.—Psoriasis on the index finger of the right hand.

PURPURA.

Definition.—Purpura may be described as a disease of the skin characterized by an effusion of red blood globules, into the cutis, and the formation of small macules varying from one-twelfth to one-half inch in diameter, usually unattended by constitutional disturbance.

Synonym.—Purples.

Symptomatology.—The spots at the time of their appearance are bright red, but gradually become purplish, and subsequently undergo the usual changes of color that are the accompaniments of a bruise. They appear mostly on the legs, and are usually symmetrically arranged; they may also show themselves on any part of the body excepting the head.

The disease occurs more in the old than in the young, and generally comes in successive crops, each crop running a course of eight or ten days. Hæmorrhage from the mucous membrane may at times complicate the trouble (*land scurvy*). It is then apt to be attended by more or less constitutional disturbance.

Treatment.—The diet should consist of the most nutritious articles. Malt preparations are useful foods. Outdoor exercise is very beneficial. Locally, hamamelis is one of the best remedies, and when there is much hæmorrhage, ice treatment may be resorted to.

Simple purpura responds best to ARSENICUM ALB., and the hæmorrhagic form to SULPHURIC ACID. Other remedies may be indicated as follows:

Aconite.—In simple cases when attended by fever.

Arnica.—Yellow, blue and reddish blue spots. In lying-in women.

BAPTISIA.—Livid spots all over the body and limbs, of the size of a three-cent piece. Great languor; desire to lie down. Tired, bruised, sick feeling all over the body.

Berberis.—Petechiæ on the right shoulder or left humerus, back of the hand and wrist. Bruised pain with stiffness and lameness in small of back. Renal or vesical complications.

BRYONIA.—Hæmorrhagic purpura. Aches and pains worse from motion. Weariness and heaviness in all the limbs. Worse when warm weather sets in after cold days.

CHLORAL.—Deep red spots on reddened bases, permanent under pressure. Hæmorrhagic purpura. Lips covered with sordes and dried blood. Great prostration.

Cocoa.—Dark spots like ecchymoses under the skin,

about the size of a pin's head, on the fingers. May be used to protect from skin diseases.

Hamamelis.—Hæmorrhagic purpura. Profuse epistaxis. Passive, venous hæmorrhages. Great lassitude and weariness. In old people.

Lachesis.—Simple purpura. Blackish-blue spots. Great physical and mental exhaustion. Climacteric troubles.

Mercurius.—Bluish-red spots, darker on the margin and lighter in the center. Increase of saliva with scorbutic gums. Tongue swollen, showing imprints of teeth on margin. Bruised feeling, with soreness in all the bones.

PHOSPHORUS.—Petechial spots on the skin. Bluish-red spots on the legs. Purple like exanthem over the whole body. Small wounds bleed much.

RRUS TOX.—Simple purpura. Dark brown spots on inside of ankles. Rheumatism of joints worse during rest. Patient changes position constantly. Swollen ankles after sitting too long. Symptoms worse in wet weather.

Terebinthina.—Hæmorrhagic purpura. Intestinal hæmorrhages. Hæmaturia. Great prostration.

Veratrum vir.—Simple purpura. Galvanic-like shocks in the limbs. Rapid pulse; slow respiration. In plethoric individuals.

RING-WORM.

Definition.—See Tricophytina.

RHINOSCLEROMA.

Definition.—Rhinoscleroma is characterized by irregularly shaped, sharp bordered, flat swellings of a normal or dark reddish-brown color, occurring for the most part on the nose and upper lip.

Symptomatology.—Rhinoscleroma is almost unknown in this country. It was first described by Hebra and Kaposi in 1870.

It is a disease of adult life, runs a slow course, and may remain stationary for years. The tubercles are seldom attended by pain, but are usually extremely sensitive to pressure.

Treatment.—When treatment is necessary the tubercles are best removed by the use of the irido-platinum points (Fig. 10) and Squibb's fused nitrate as recommended in Lupus vulgaris.

Calcarea phos. will probably be the most useful internal remedy. Guaraca, and Rhus rad., may be studied.

RODENT ULCER.

Definition.—See Epithelioma.

ROSACEA.

Definition.—Rosacea is a chronic disease, affecting more particularly the nose, cheeks and forehead, resulting from a dilatation of the blood vessels with increased growth of connective tissue, and characterized by redness and a tendency to the development of tubercles and pustules.

Symptomatology.—Rosacea has three stages. In the

first there is more or less passive hyperæmia of the parts affected. The whole diseased surface may be reddened, or it may be reddened only in spots. If the nose is attacked, it is apt to feel cold and greasy to the touch. After months or perhaps years, the *second* stage sets in. The redness is now more marked, and minute blood-vessels appear upon the surface. As the disease progresses these vessels increase in size, and take a tortuous course. Sooner or later, the integument becomes thickened, acne papules and pustules show themselves, the nose becomes warm, and the disease passes into the *third* stage.

It may remain in this condition for years, or if the morbid action continues, great thickening and hypertrophy of the parts, with deformity may result.

Etiology.—It is mostly a disease of middle life. It attacks both sexes, but males more than females. Anything which tends to increase the circulation in the face may produce rosacea. Excessive spirituous indulgence is a prominent cause, as is also functional or organic disease of the uterus or ovaries.

Prognosis.—The prognosis is generally favorable if the disease has not passed beyond the first stage.

Treatment.—In the first stage a sulphur lotion one (4.) to three drachms (12.) to the ounce (32.) of lavender water, may be used with benefit.

In the second stage the distended blood-vessels should be incised bi-weekly. Gossypium may be used to check the hæmorrhage. Good results are obtained from single or multiple punctures of the vessels with a fine cambric needle attached to the negative pole of a galvanic battery, with from six to ten elements in the circuit.

As a last resort, portions of the redundant integument may be excised, or erased with the dermal curette (Fig. 9).

The internal remedy will usually be one of the following:

Agaricus.—Redness with burning heat in the face. Burning itching on the cheeks. In drunkards and after sexual debauches.

Antimonium crud.—Red points with white dots in the center. Thick white coating on the tongue. Gastric derangements.

Arsenicum alb.—In long-lasting cases with debility. Rough, dirty looking skin. Burning itching, painful after scratching.

ARSENICUM BROMIDE.—Violet papules on the nose.

Arsenicum iodide.—Redness with itching. In scrofulous subjects.

BELLADONNA.—Nose red, swollen and shining, with small red pimples. Great dryness of the nose. Swelling and tension of the upper lip. Parts feel hot to the touch. In plethoric subjects.

Bromine.—Pimples on the nose. Soreness under the nose and on margins of nostrils. Swelling of the thyroid gland. In light-haired persons.

Calcium sulphide.—When there is a pustular tendency.

Calcarea phos.—Nose shining like oil. Heartburn with other gastric symptoms after dinner.

Cannabis.—Large pimples surrounded by red swelling. Aggravation in the morning, with burning like fire. Urinary complications.

Carbo animalis.—Pimples on the face. Eruption like red spots on the cheeks. Morning nose-bleed preceded by vertigo. Eructations tasting of food eaten long before. In scrofulous, venous constitutions.

Causticum.—Pimples on the nose. Tendency to ulceration.

Curare.—Pimples like tubercles on the tip of the nose. Rosacea with varices and bleeding of the cheeks.

Guarea trich.—Rosacea with pains as from excoriation when touched.

Hydrocotyle.—Papular eruption on the face. Tickling in the nose.

Nux juglans.—In strumous subjects.

Nux vom.—Rosacea associated with dyspepsia and constipation. In drunkards.

Opium.—Dusky red bloated appearance.

Phosphorus.—Pimples on the face and wing of the nose.

Petroleum.—In the second stage. Parts very painful to slight touch. Nausea from riding in a carriage or ship.

Rhus rad.—Tip of the nose red and painful, as if it would suppurate.

Ruta.—Rosacea. Deep fine stitches in the parts. Aggravated by eating uncooked food.

Sulphur.—In chronic cases.

ROSEOLA.

Definition.—See Erythema.

RUPIA.

Definition.—Rupia may be the result of either the pustular or the bullous syphilide. It consists of thick, greenish or blackish "cockle-shaped" crusts, covering unhealthy punched-out looking ulcers. It is a late and malignant manifestation of syphilis, and is seldom met with in private practice.

Treatment.—MERCURIUS BIJODAT., and *Potassium iodide*, are the principal internal remedies. Arsenicum, Berberis aqu., and Nit. acid may be studied. Locally, iodide of starch dressings are serviceable.

SALT-RHEUM.

Definition.—See Eczema.

SARCOMA CUTIS.

Definition.—Sarcoma cutis consists of brownish-red, variously sized tubercles or nodules, attended by a diffused thickening of the skin. It is a rare and malignant disease, occurs mostly in adult life, and usually terminates fatally.

SCABIES.

Definition.—Scabies is a contagious disease caused by the burrowing of an animal parasite called the *acarus scabiei*, in the skin, and is characterized by the formation of *cuniculi* attended with intense nightly itching and having as accidental accompaniments, vesicles, pustules and crusts.

Synonym.—The itch.

Symptomatology.—The first symptom after exposure to the contagion, is usually a more or less extensive local irritation of the skin, attended by the formation of minute inflammatory points or vesicles, and an itching characteristically worse at night. On examining the parts carefully at this stage, a burrow or cuniculus, just beneath the horny layer, may be discovered as a slightly raised, straight or tortuous line, with a vesicle at one end, and the itch insect marked by a whitish-yellow speck, headed off by a dark curved line, at the other. The disease spreads from this point, usually with great rapidity, so that in four or six weeks it may cover the greater part of the body. The parts most obnoxious to this affection are, in adults the interdigits, the front of the arm and wrists, the flexures of the joints and the dorsal surface of the penis. In children the buttocks and ankles are as a rule primarily affected oftener than the other parts. The disease seldom appears above the nipple line, and in chronic cases is found more on the abdomen and inner surface of the upper part of the thigh.

The vesicles are generally isolated, irregular in size and shape, stand out prominently, and are frequently topped with short burrows. On acount of the intense itching, "scratch-marks" may so mask the disease as to at times, almost obliterate the cuniculi and vesicles. These "scratch-marks" are, however, in their turn, more or less characteristic of scabies.

The cause of scabies is the *acarus scabiei.* The disease arises only from contagion. It may be conveyed from one person to another by hand shaking or by sleeping with one who is affected. All are subject to the contagion, whether high or low, rich or poor. Men are as a rule oftener affected than women. It is one of the more common skin diseases in Europe, but in this country it is quite rare.

The acarus exists male and female, and is barely visible to the naked eye, being about half a millimeter in length. To the zoologist it is a beautiful and elegant little creature. It resembles a turtle in shape, and has an oval body, convex on the back, and flat on the belly. The back is armed with short spines, which are directed backwards, and are so arranged as to effectually thwart any attempt at retrogression on the part of the insect. The head is small and closely set to the body, and is devoid of eyes. There are four front legs armed with suckers, and four hind legs armed with hairs. The two inner hind legs in the male are armed with suckers. The organs of generation are conspicuously marked on the under surface of the body. The female acarus is thrice the size of the male. Males are short lived. The female lives from three to four months, and lays from 24 to 50 eggs at the rate of from one to two a day. As the male insect is seldom found on the skin, it is presumed that he plays but an inferior part in the development of scabies.

The female acarus within thirty minutes after its arrival on the skin, commences boring perpendicularly through the horny layer and tunnels a place in which to lay its eggs. This burrow or tunnel is called a cuniculus, and may vary from two to several centimeters in length. Here is the little miner's habitat, in which the deposited eggs are usually hatched in about two weeks. The young acari or "brigands" as they are sometimes called, are liberated in the order of their birth, by the gradual wearing off of the horny layer of the cuticle, and most invariably adopt the mining habits of their progenitors.

The acarus has considerable tenacity of life. It has been known to live from eight to ten days in water, and from two to four days in vinegar.

Diagnosis.—The following are the main diagnostic points of scabies:

1. The presence of cuniculi with their contained acari.

2. The seat of the eruption, which is mostly in the interdigits and wrists, and in the flexures of the body, the buttocks, and on the dorsal surface of the penis. Scabies seldom appears above the nipple line.

3. The multiformity of the eruption.

4. The itching, which though continuing through the day is characteristically worse at night.

5. The evidences of contagion in the household, other members of the family being affected.

6. The rapid disappearance of all the symptoms under parasiticidal treatment.

Prognosis.—The prognosis may usually be considered favorable, provided a correct diagnosis is made, otherwise the disease may last for years.

Treatment.—Once recognized the disease is speedily cured. A high potency of *Sulphur* given internally has the reputation of curing scabies, but perhaps the best and most prompt results will be had from well directed local treatment, as the disappearance of the trouble depends on the removal of the cause, or in other words, upon the death of the insect.

Sulphur ointment—one (4.) to two drachms (8.) to the ounce (32.)—is to be recommended as the best parasiticide. Storax ointment is preferred by some, as being cheaper and less liable to irritate the skin. (Care must always be taken in using parasiticides not to have them too strong, as the secondary rash is invariably aggravated thereby.) The Oil of lavender may at times be used, as may also the Balsam of Peru.

Before using the parasiticide, the patient should be ordered to take a hot soap and water bath. The cerate or oil may then be rubbed firmly into the skin of the *whole* body for twenty minutes, and allowed to remain on all night. In the morning another hot soap and water bath should be taken. The same programme may be followed on the next and succeeding evenings, or until every trace of itching is gone. In this way the majority of cases of itch can be cured in from one to three days. All the clothing of the patient should be carefully boiled or baked before being used.

SCLERODERMA.

Definition.—Scleroderma is a chronic affection characterized by hardness and inelasticity of the integument.

Synonym.—Hide bound skin.

Symptomatology.—It is a rare disease, and commonly commences as a circumscribed infiltration of the skin and subcutaneous tissues. As the disease advances, the parts are found to become hard and immovable, as if *frozen* or *petrified.* The skin has generally a yellowish-brown or at times waxy appearance. Scleroderma may occur on any part of the body, and at any period of life, and is apt to be symmetrical. It is supposed to be due to a stagnation of lymph in the lymph spaces. It runs a chronic course, but tends to get well in years.

Diagnosis.—The disease bears some resemblance to morphœa, with which it is apt to be confounded. Scleroderma, however, is pathologically a hypertrophy, while morphœa is an atrophy.

Treatment.—Galvanism is recommended as having proved beneficial in some cases. As internal remeuies, *Antimonium crudum*, Alumina, Berberis, Eiæis and Rhus tox., may be studied.

SCLERIASIS.

Definition.—Scleriasis is an induration of the cellular tissue in new born children.

Symptomatology.—It may be congenital or appear during the first months of infant life. The skin which is at first of a yellowish, brownish or reddish hue, gradually fades and becomes hard and rigid. The surface is generally cold, and more or less œdema is usually present.

Etiology.—The causes of this disease are supposed to be congenital debility, vascular disturbances and affections of the navel. The inflexibility is caused by a stearine-like deposit in the subcutaneous tissue.

Prognosis.—The prognosis is unfavorable, as most children die with some affection of the lungs.

Treatment.—*Elœis guineensis* may prove useful as an internal remedy. Hydrocotyle, Phosphorus and Stillingia may be thought of.

SCROFULODERMA.

Definition.—Scrofuloderma is a strumous disease of the skin, commencing as indolent, painless livid tubercles that slowly soften and give place to unhealthy ulcers with free incrustation.

Symptomatology.—It is oftenest encountered on the neck, and beneath the lower jaw, but is frequently met with on the thorax, and in the axillæ and groins. The cause of this disease is to be found in that peculiar condition of system, which has been termed scrofulosis.

Diagnosis.—It is to be differentiated from syphilis, lupus, and epithelioma.

Treatment.—Such patients should be allowed an abundance of fresh air, plenty of outdoor exercise, and a generous diet. Cod liver oil should be one of their standard foods. Locally, the ulcers when formed may be dressed with the *iodide of starch* paste.

The CALCIUM SULPHIDE, is the principal internal remedy.

The Calcium iodide, Theridion, and Scrofularia may be compared.

SEBACEOUS CYST.

Definition.—A sebaceous cyst is a whitish round or oval tumor of variable size, composed of sebaceous matter enclosed in a sac.

Synonym.—Wen.

Symptomatology.—The tumors occur either singly or in numbers, and appear mostly on the scalp, face and back. Their contents are either hard and friable, soft and cheesy, or fluid in character. They are usually painless, run a chronic course, and may end spontaneously by degeneration of the contents and destruction of the cyst.

Treatment.—Excision is the best local remedy. POTASSIUM IODIDE 1x, *Baryta carb.*, and Bromine, have more or less repute in removing cysts, and may be used to prevent their return.

SEBORRHŒA.

Definition.—Seborrhœa is a functional disorder of the sebaceous glands, characterized by an excessive secretion of sebum.

Synonyms.—Steatorrhœa. Sebaceous flux.

Symptomatology.—It may appear on any portion of the body, but attacks chiefly the scalp and face. It occurs at all periods of life, is seen more in women than in men, and is either local or general. In the newly-born it is a physiological rather than a pathological process, and constitutes the *vernix caseosa.* As a disease it appears either in the form of an oily coating on the skin, or as dirty-white or yellow flat scales, which are more or less greasy, and slightly adherent (*dandruff*). Light complexioned people are more subject to the former, and dark complexioned to the latter.

When occurring on the scalp, seborrhœa is one of the most frequent causes of baldness; and as a sequel of variola an oily nose is not uncommon.

Diagnosis.—This affection may at times be very easily confounded with eczema. But if it is remembered that seborrhœa is always a dry or oily disease, and that eczema has always a history of discharge; and also that the scales of seborrhœa are usually seated on a pale bluish-colored skin, and abundant, while those of eczema are scanty and seated on a reddened more or less infiltrated surface, the diagnosis will not be difficult.

Treatment.—The hygienic influences should be so arranged as to keep the system in the healthiest possible state. All oily scales and crusts should be saturated with some oily substance, such as olive oil or glycerine, before their removal is attempted. Ten or twelve hours generally suffices to macerate them, so that they can be readily removed with warm soap and water. The common hard soap is scarcely strong enough for this purpose, and so sapo viridis should be used. An elegant preparation is made by mixing four drachms (16.) of sapo viridis with three drachms (12.) of cologne water. After this treatment one of the simple oils should be applied, otherwise the skin will become dry and harsh.

In mild cases all the local treatment that is necessary is an infusion of saponaria bark applied morning and evening.

For seborrhœa occurring on the face, a tannin dusting powder prepared by mixing from twenty grains (1.3) to one drachm (4.) of tannic acid with one ounce (32.) of rice powder, has been highly recommended.

The most serviceable internal remedies are the following:

Arsenicum alb.—Smutty brown, mottled skin. Yellow color of face.

Ammonium mur.—Large accumulation of bran-like scales, with falling off of the hair.

BUFO.—Skin greenish, and always looking dirty and oily.

BRYONIA.—In long lasting cases.

Calcarea carb.—Nose shines as from oil. Seborrhœa with hyperæmia of the scalp and headache.

Graphites.—Seborrhœa behind the ears.

Iodine.—Firmly adhering scales, which leave the skin red and painful, on removal.

Kali carb.—Dry hair rapidly falling off, with much dandruff.

Lycopodium.—Seborrhœa on the chin.

Mercurius sol.—Seborrhœa of the genitals, accompanied with hyperæmia.

Mezereum.—Excessive formation of smegma.

NATRUM MUR.—Severe itching of the scalp. The hair falls out in masses. Seborrhœa of the face.

PLUMBUM.—The skin of the face shines as if oily, and feels oily.

Phosphorus.—Copious dandruff; falls off in clouds.

Potassium bromide.—Seborrhœa on hairy portions of the face, forehead and neck.

Raphanus.—Skin is greasy and makes the hands greasy to touch it.

Sepia.—Seborrhœa of the genitals in women.

Sulphur.—Dandruff.

Thuja.—White scaly dandruff. Hair dry and falling off.

Vinca minor.—Seborrhœa on upper lip and base of the nose.

SHINGLES.

Definition.—See Zoster.

STROPHULUS.

Definition.—Strophulus is a disease of early life, due to congestion about the mouths of the sweat follicles, and is characterized by the appearance of small red or white papules, varying in size from a pin's head to a millet seed.

Synonyms.—Red-gum. Tooth rash.

Symptomatology.—The face, neck and arms are the usual seats of the eruption, but it may be general in its distribution. There are two forms of the affection. One variety mostly due to over-clothing, appears in infants a few weeks old. In this the eruption reaches its height in two or three days, and then gradually disappears. The other variety is frequently met with during the period of dentition, lasts longer than the former variety, and is often associated with gastro-intestinal disturbance.

Treatment.—The diet should be carefully regulated, and all superfluous clothing abandoned. Lancing the gums is proper only when they are swollen or so tender as to distress the child.

CHAMOMILLA is the principal internal remedy. *Calcarea carb.* may be called for when there is a chronic acidity. Spiranthes is often indicated. *Borax*, *Ledum*, Apis, Cicuta, and Sumbul, may be studied.

SUDAMINA.

Definition.—Sudamina is a disorder of the sweat glands, characterized by pin-head sized vesicles formed by the collection of sweat between the layers of the epidermis.

Symptomatology.—It is more particularly met with during the summer months, and in acute febrile and constitutional diseases. It occurs both in children and adults, and may be esteemed a sign of general debility. The mal-administration of Turkish baths occasionally gives rise to a general attack.

Treatment.—BRYONIA, *Ammonium mur.*, and Urtica urens, are the most important remedies.

SYCOSIS.

Definition.—Sycosis is a catarrhal inflammation of the hair follicles of the beard, and is characterized by the formation of papules, tubercles and pustules, attended with pain, heat and swelling.

Synonyms.—Mentagra. Folliculitis pilorum.

Symptomatology.—The affection demonstrates itself by the development of acuminated, more or less indurated, pin-head or split-pea sized pustules immediately around the hairs, containing a thick yellow fluid. More or less peri-follicular inflammation usually accompanies the disease, and according as this is slight or severe, the patient suffers pain. If the inflammation is severe the pustules are crowded together, otherwise they are generally discrete. The hairs of the affected part are as a rule healthy, and cause pain on extraction (a characteristic). The disease is not contagious.

Treatment.—Shaving is the first thing to be done, and it must, if necessary, be kept up daily for months. Hot fomentations should be applied if there is much inflammation.

As regards the internal treatment, TARTAR EMET., is allowed by common consent to rank first. Other remedies occasionally of service, are:

CALCIUM SULPHIDE.—Many little pimples on the chin, sore when touched. Large sores surrounded by small pustules. Œdematous swelling of the parts.

CEREUS SERPENTINUS.—Pustules on the right upper lip and angle of the mouth, on parts covered by beard. Itching of the parts covered by the beard.

Cicuta.—Elevated eruption which causes burning pain when touched. Itching papular eruption on chin.

Graphites.—Chin covered with eruption. Hard white pimples on red base. Dry skin; never perspires. Worse on the left side.

Kali bich.—Pustules on the right side of the chin,

seated on reddened bases. In fat, light-haired persons.

MERCURIUS PRECIP. RUBER is, next to Tartar emet., one of the most prompt remedies for sycosis.

Petroleum.—Papular eruption at the corner of the mouth with sticking pain. Painful pustules on the chin.

Sulphur.—Painful pea-sized pimples, with red areolæ.

SYPHILIDES.

Definition.—Syphilides are the manifestations of general syphilis upon the skin.

Symptomatology.—They may be divided into two arbitrary groups, viz., the *secondary* and the *tertiary;* and possess the following general features:

They have a history of syphilitic inoculation. They are of a reddish, yellow-brown color, often described as copper-colored. They are polymorphous and elective. They are devoid of both pain and itching. The crusts are thick, greenish-black. The ulcers are of an ash-gray color, are often serpiginous or horse-shoe shaped, and are bounded by sharply cut edges. The diffused eruptions are generally symmetrical. Later the distribution is irregular. The scales occur in small circular spots, and are thinner and fewer in number than in non-syphilitic cases. They are of a non-inflammatory character and are prone to recur. They occur in the ratio of about five per cent. of all cutaneous cases.

The SECONDARY SYPHILIDES are:

1. *Erythematous syphilide.*—This consists in the

formation of flat or slightly raised patches, varying in size from a split pea to a two-cent piece. It is the earliest and most frequent cutaneous manifestation of constitutional syphilis, and appears generally at about the sixth week. It often comes on slowly, but may appear suddenly, and is confined in the majority of cases, to the covered parts of the body. When it occurs early in the disease it may last for months. The rash is unaccompanied by itching, but is usually attended by such significant signs of syphilis, as the chancre or its scar, the redness of the fauces, and the mucous patches.

Treatment.—The white precipitate ointment, ten (.6) to twenty grains (1.3) to the ounce (32.), may be used externally, and MERC. IODAT., or MERC. COR., given at the same time internally.

2. *Papular syphilide.*—This eruption is usually superficial and may either follow the former, or occur as the first outbreak after chancre. It may appear as early as the third week after the chancre, or not until the fourth month, and usually lasts from three to eight weeks. The papules may be either acuminated or broad and flattened, and may vary in size from a millet seed to a split pea or larger. They are at first rose-colored, and are surrounded by a white border of fine scales. Later they assume a tawny hue, and may be moist, or covered with thin scales. They are usually most marked on the nape of the neck, the flexor surfaces of the extremities, and on the perineum and genitals.

Treatment.—The five per cent. oleate of mercury is the best local application. Internally, POTASSIUM IODIDE and *Merc. cor.* are the principal remedies.

3. *Vesicular syphilide.*—This is a rare type of syphilitic eruption, and in the majority of cases, takes the form of *herpes.* Occasionally it is *varicellaform.*

The vesicles of the *herpetic* manifestation vary in size from a millet seed to a pea, and are seated upon a copper colored base. They are arranged either in circles or in segments of circles, usually last about a week, and disappear without scarring. Their first appearance is generally about three weeks after the disappearance of the primary lesion.

The vesicles of the *varicellaform* eruption are about the size of small peas, are surrounded by a coppery-red areola, and are now and then umbilicated. They may be either isolated or confluent, and are succeeded by greenish-brown scabs which fall off in about two weeks, leaving slowly disappearing purplish discolorations. The lesion appears about the sixth month after chancre, and shows itself mostly about the face.

Treatment.—MERC. COR., *Cinnabar*, and Merc. jodatus are three main internal remedies. A Merc. cor. lotion or the oleate of mercury, may be used externally.

4. *Pigmentary syphilide.*—This consists of "coffee-with-milk" colored macules, varying in size from a cent piece to a half dollar. It occurs oftenest in women, and appears mostly on the neck, but occasionally extends to the body and extremities. It comes

between the fourth and twelfth month, and lasts one or two months, or longer.

Treatment.—NITRIC ACID is the generally indicated remedy. The *Calcium sulphide* is sometimes called for.

5. *Pustular syphilide.*—This may exist in either of three forms:

(*a.*) As small millet-seed sized ephemeral dead-gray colored pustules which dry up and form brownish, rough, scabs, or else linger as slightly ulcerating, vegetating surfaces. They are apt to appear on the forehead, angles of the mouth and base of the nose, and usually leave a brownish centrally depressed spot on their disappearance.

(*b.*) As pin-head or split-pea sized acuminated pustules which form brownish colored scabs, and leave small, white, depressed cicatrices. They develop about six months after chancre, and last about two months. They appear mostly on the scalp, face, and trunk, and more rarely on the lower extremities.

(*c.*) As ecthymatous umbilicated pustules, which vary in size from a pea to a hickory nut, and are surrounded by a dark areola. These form rough, dark, greenish-brown scabs, and leave slight copper-colored cicatrices, which gradually disappear.

Treatment.—Locally, white precipitate ointment may be used.

KALI BICH. and *Merc. nit.* are the more common internal remedies.

6. *Bullous syphilide.*—The eruption is character-

ized by blebs, which vary in size from a pea to a walnut, and after lasting a variable time, dry up and form dark greenish-brown scabs. It is a rare and late manifestation of syphilis, but may occur on the palms and soles of the newly-born as a result of inherited disease.

Treatment.—POTASSIUM IODIDE and *Syphilinum*, are the generally used remedies.

7. *Squamous syphilide.*—This may develop on the syphilized, in the course of other eruptions, or start as a primary condition with febrile symptoms, by the formation of small, red, circular blotches, which in a few days become covered with scales. After a few weeks the scales fall off, leaving dark colored spots, that gradually disappear without cicatrization.

Lentil-sized, copper colored spots, sometimes form on the palms of the hands and soles of the feet. The patches may be either fissured, or covered by adherent grayish scales, and are usually limited by the characteristic livid areola.

The eruption is commonly symmetrical, and may last for months, or even years. The scaly syphilides rarely appear before the sixth month from the chancre, and when entirely removed by treatment are not apt to return.

Treatment.—The local treatment consists in the use of the red precipitate ointment.

The internal remedies are MERC. PRECIP. RUBER. *Arsenicum sulphide* and *Cinnabar*, Sarsaparilla, Merc. cor., and Phytolacca.

8. *Tubercular syphilide.*—This is a common form

of secondary syphilis verging on the tertiary. It rarely appears before a year or longer after chancre, and consists of circumscribed, dome-shaped, brownish-red elevations, which vary in size from a split pea to a nut. They are situated for the most part on the face and back, but occasionally appear on the extremities. They develop slowly, may last for weeks or months, and disappear either by absorption or ulceration. When absorption takes place, small depressed pigmented spots remain, which either finally disappear or leave but very superficial cicatrices.

If ulceration ensues, the tubercles become covered with a brownish or blackish crust, and the ulcers have a punched-out appearance. Occasionally the eruption is grouped into circles or figures-of-eight, a peculiarity observed mostly about the forehead and nose.

Treatment.—The tubercles may be treated locally with the acid nitrate of mercury, and when ulcers form they may be dressed with iodide of starch paste.

MERC. BINIOD , and *Potassium iodide* are the generally indicated remedies. Thuja is adapted to mucous tubercles.

THE TERTIARY SYPHILIDES are principally *Rupia* and the *Gummatous syphilide.*

9. *Gummatous syphilide.*—This is a late syphilide, and appears first as little hard lumps, seldom larger than a hazel-nut situated on the head, buttocks and flexor surfaces of the extremities. They are loosely imbedded in the tissues, may be either single or multiple and grow slowly. They either undergo absorp-

tion or eventually break down, and form grayish deeply excavated ulcers that vary in size from a finger nail to the palm of the hand.

Treatment.—In addition to the treatment suggested for the eighth syphilide, CARBO ANIMALIS, Condurango, Berberis aqui, and Bi-cyanide of Mercury may be thought of. In mercurio-syphilitic ulcers, Cistus canadensis acts well.

SYPHILIDES IN CHILDREN.—The cutaneous manifestations of *hereditary syphilis*, as observed in children, differ from those of the acquired form as seen in the syphilized adult. Usually within two or three weeks after the birth of the tainted child, distinctive signs of syphilization show themselves. The little one, hitherto, it may be, of robust appearance, gradually declines in health. Fissures and chaps appear about the mouth, anus and genitals. The skin becomes harsh and dry and assumes a dingy, yellowish hue. The face grows wrinkled, and the babe patient appears like a little dried up old man. Sooner or later snuffles sets in, the disease extends to the larynx, and the child has a peculiar hoarse cry. About the same time coppery-red mucous patches varying in size from a finger-nail to the palm of the hand, appear on the buttocks, thighs or genitals. Occasionally the hands exfoliate in thin dry scales. After a variable season, dry or moist papules—the moist predominating—make their appearance on the reddened patches. Tubercles may form. The matrix of the nail may suppurate and the nail be shed several times. *Excoria-*

tions and *mucous patches* are the most common, and at the same time, the most characteristic manifestations of syphilis in the young. Occasionally syphilis is acquired by a healthy baby from nursing a woman with chancre, or through vaccination. This is called *Infantile syphilis*. If the child is born with a general eruption, death is almost inevitable. The bullous syphilide in infants usually manifests itself at birth, and generally results fatally.

Treatment.—The CALCIUM IODIDE is the principal remedy, and next Merc. viv. *Corallium rub.*, is adapted to the syphilitic erosions. A five per cent. oleate of mercury inunction is highly recommended. If the simple oleate irritates the skin, equal parts of a ten per cent. oleate and vaseline may be used. One-half of a drachm of the unguent may be used at each application.

TELANGIECTASIS.

Definition.—Telangiectasis is characterized by circumscribed, vascular cutaneous growths, appearing for the most part during adult life.

Synonyms.—Spider nævus.

Symptomatology.—The growths are usually of a bright red color, and vary in size from a pin's head to a split pea. They differ from nævi in that they are not congenital, but acquired. Telangiectasis selects as its favorite seats the face and neck. It runs a chronic course, and may either terminate spontaneously or remain through life.

Treatment.—The treatment is the same as that of nævus.

CONDURANGO is reported as having cured some cases.

THE TINEÆ.

Definition.—"The tineæ" is a generic term given to a class of cutaneous affections that owe their origin to vegetable parasites.

Symptomatology.—At the Central Homœopathic Dispensary they constitute about four per cent. of all the cases in the department for skin diseases. They are all contagious, occur more in populous districts, and are curable by parasiticides.

Parasites.—The parasites are the *Achorion Schonleinii*, the *Tricophyton* and the *Microsporon furfur*. They exist in three forms:

1. *Conidia* or *spores*, which are made up of an outer and inner enveloping membrane composed of cellulose, enclosing a liquid containing floating granules. They present an average diameter of .006 mm.

2. *Mycelia*, or thread-like structures, which vary in size and shape from simple, fine, transparent filaments, to large, double-contoured tubes.

3. *Granules*, the nuclear form of the fully developed fungus. They require a high power for their detection.

The conidia are the most developed parts of the fungus. They may be either round or oval. The mycelia are the growing or producing structures. They may be either long or short, branched or straight, filled with or almost devoid of granules; and the granules being the more elementary forms, may be either numerous or only sparcely distributed.

From this it may be noted, that whenever in the field of the microscope, a large number of conidia or spores are seen it can be safely said that the fungus has age, and that consequently the disease has been running for some time, or has become *chronic.* If on the other hand sprouting mycelia filled with granules, marked off as it were by partitions, and called *sporophores*, are present in large numbers, it may be taken for granted that the fungus growth is active, and that consequently the disease is spreading rapidly, or is in the *acute* stage.

Varieties of Tineæ.—There are three varieties of "*the tineæ*," due respectively to the ravages committed by the afore-mentioned parasites upon the skin.

They are *Tinea favosa*, *Tinea tricophytina* and *Tinea versicolor*.

TINEA FAVOSA.

Definition.—Tinea favosa is a contagious disease, characterized by the presence of one or more clustered or scattered variously sized cup-shaped scabs of a sulphur-yellow color, and pierced by a hair.

Synonyms.—Favus. Crusted ringworm. Honey-combed ringworm.

Symptomatology.—It appears mostly among the poorer classes and flourishes in dirt. It is oftenest found on the head, frequently on the trunk, and occasionally on the lower extremities. It shows itself first at the point where the vegetable parasite touches the skin, as a slight redness, accompanied by a varying amount of itching. Scales soon make their appearance on the reddened surface and assume the form of pin-head sized crusts. These continue to increase, and the disease spreads, so that at the end of two weeks, the collected mass presents the umbilicated form of the fully developed favus cup. They may now remain separated, or coalesce and form yellowish-colored, aggregations, having a characteristic honeycomb aspect.

The scabs are peculiarly cup-shaped in appearance, with the concavity directed upwards, and vary in size from a split pea to a ten cent piece or even larger. They have a straw or sulphur-yellow color, and are as a rule pierced by a hair. A special odor generally attaches to the favus crust; it is that of stale straw, mice or cat's urine.

On removing the scab, the skin is seen to present a more or less reddened, hollowed out appearance, corresponding to the convexity on its under surface.

Most generally the hair is loosened in the follicle, by the fungus affecting its formative apparatus, and comes away with the scab. If the disease is severe, and the ravages of the parasite are in any way extensive, the hair follicles may be destroyed and the scalp left red, smooth and shining. Favus may, at least in this country, be classed among the rarer diseases. It is eminently contagious, never originates spontaneously, but may be communicated from animals to man. It may have its seat in either the hair follicles or the hair, or upon the surface of the skin, and is due to the action of the vegetable parasite known as the *achorion schonleinii.* This fungus was named after Schonlein, its discoverer, by Remy. Its history dates back to 1839. Under the microscope it presents the following characteristics:

A field studded mostly with *oval* conidia, varied as to size, and mycelia variable as to length and more or less filled with granules. The oval fungus has a double envelope, and an average diameter of .034 mm. The mycelia present a pale grayish watery appearance, and have an average diameter of .0026 mm. They—the mycelia—are usually abundant, and occasionally assume a peculiar grouping with the conidia. (I allude to the clustering of four or five of the spores in a row at the end of a mycelial thread.) This is oftener found than many would have us believe, and when present is characteristic of favus.

Diagnosis.—As regards the diagnosis of tinea favosa, little difficulty is usually experienced. Briefly, the distinguishing points are:

The characteristic pea-sized, straw-colored, cup-shaped, honey-combed crusts. The stale straw odor. Its prevalence among the poorer classes and children. The presence of the achorion schonleinii, as revealed by the microscope. Its contagiousness.

From eczema, for which it is most liable to be mistaken, it may be distinguished by having no stage of discharge, by having sulphur-yellow instead of greenish-yellow crusts; by its stale straw odor, as contrasted with the nauseous smell of eczema; by being contagious, and eczema not; and by being cured by parasiticides, while eczema would be aggravated thereby.

Treatment.—The cardinal point in the treatment, is either to starve out or kill the parasite. The former may be accomplished by the administration of internal remedies which may so alter the soil as to render it less suitable to the fructification of the plant, and the latter by the use of local applications, called parasiticides. Before local treatment is commenced, all crusts must be removed and the diseased hairs pulled out. Almond oil, a marsh-mallow, or mashed turnip poultice, will soften the crusts. The hairs are best removed by a broad-lipped epilation forceps. (Fig. 12). After the scabs and diseased hairs have been

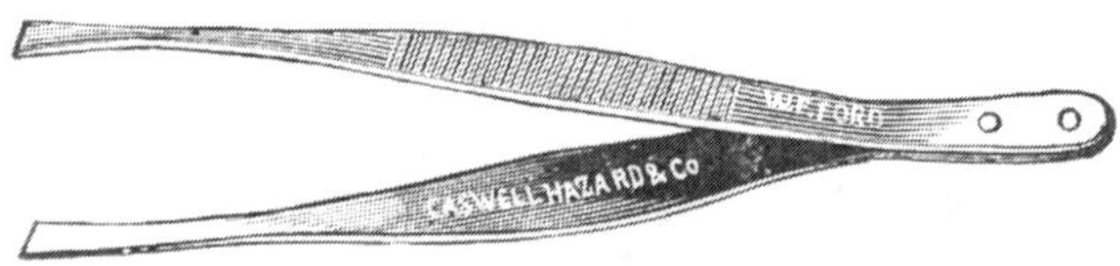

FIG 12. EPILATING FORCEPS.

removed, a parasiticide of greater or less strength, depending upon the irritability of the skin and the stubbornness of the parasite, should be applied. A mercuric bichloride lotion—one (.06) to three grains (.19) to the ounce (32.)—acts well. If the fungus has caused considerable irritation, enough over and above the scabbing to occasion a discharge, the oleate of mercury five per cent will be of service. Care must be taken in using parasiticides not to have them too strong, otherwise more harm than good may result from their use.

Of internal remedies the following may be mentioned:

Agaricus.—Favus with biting itching in the scalp. Crusts sometimes spread to other parts of the body. Sensation as if ice-cold needles were piercing the skin.

Arsenicum iodide.—Scalp dry and rough, and covered with dry scales and scabs. Extend to forehead, face and ears. Intense itching and burning.

BROMINE.—In children with light hair and blue eyes. When the fungus excites considerable irritation of the skin. Profuse dirty looking, offensive smelling discharge. Crawling beneath the skin of the occiput.

Calcarea carb.—Thick scabs covering a quantity of thick yellow pus. Large scabs, covering sometimes over one-half the entire scalp. Burning and itching. Glandular swellings on the neck. In fair, plump children.

Dulcamara.—In scrofulous children when the crusts are thick and the hair falls out. Bleeding after scratching. Glandular swellings in the neighborhood of the eruption.

Graphites.—Exudation of clear, glutinous fluid forming moist scabs. Secretion from scratching. Falling out of hair. Skin dry and inclined to crack. Tendency to ulceration.

KALI CARB.—Exudation of moisture after scratching. Sensitiveness to cold. Frequent urination, especially at night. Dryness and falling out of the hair. In old over-treated cases.

Lappa major.—Grayish-white, foul smelling crusts. Most of the hair has disappeared. Swelling and suppuration of the axillary glands. Boils all over the body.

Lycopodium.—Eruption beginning on the back of the head. When there are several spots, and when the crusts are fetid, thick and bleed easily. Hunger, but a small quantity of food fills him up. Constipation.

Mezereum.—Elevated white chalk-like scabs with ichor beneath, breeding vermin. Itching as if the head were in an ant's nest. Worse at night. In scrofulous children.

Oleander.—Favus on the back part of the head and behind the ears. Biting itching of the scalp as from vermin. Skin sensitive and sore.

Phosphorus.—May be used when the follicles appear to have been destroyed, and the scalp left smooth and shining.

Sulphur.—May be necessary to help along the action of the indicated drug.

Ustilago mad.—When there is great moisture, with matting and falling of the hair.

Vinca minor.—Offensive, moist eruption with brownish crusts. Abundance of lice on the head. Hair matted together. The hair falls out in single spots and white hairs grow there.

Viola tricolor.—Thick crusts; hair becomes matted; urine smells like cat's urine. Swelling of the cervical glands. Intolerable itching at night.

TINEA TRICOPHYTINA.

Definition.—Tinea tricophytina is the variety of tinea that owes its origin to the tricophyton.

Synonyms.—Ringworm. Barber's itch.

Symptomatology.—Under this head are included the diseases commonly described as, tinea tonsurans, tinea circinnata, tinea sycosis, and tinea kerion. The tricophyton finds its affinity in children of lymphatic temperament, selects as its seat either the scalp or body, and there produces the disease known by the common name, "ringworm." In middle life it frequently attacks the beard, where it grows luxuriantly and causes the affection having the vernacular "barber's itch."

When the fungus is first planted on the skin, the fates being propitious, it demonstrates its presence as does the favus fungus by the appearance of an itching erythematous redness, accompanied usually by a crop of evanescent vesicles, which are quickly followed by a scaly formation.

If the parasite attacks the scalp, it will be noticed that the hairs covering the patch or patches, gradually become brittle and break off, or are loosened and come out easily. The breaking off of the hairs gives to an old patch a "stubble-like" appearance, which together with a semblance of "goose-skin," due to the prominence of the follicles, may be held as characteristic.

On the body, where it presents its best developed ringworm appearance, tinea tricophytina spreads in a circular fairy-ring-like manner, until it covers an area of a silver dollar or even larger. For, as the skin becomes accustomed to the presence of the fungus which has already assumed the cellular form in the oldest part of the patch, the central redness gradually fades, while the disease is all the time spreading in the direction of the periphery, where the sprouting mycelia are most active. When the parasite attacks the beard, a slight inflammation is first noticed around one or more hair follicles of the chin, which gradually increases until papules make their appearance. The papules steadily enlarge, so that in about a week's time they may have reached the size of split peas or hazel-nuts, and have in fact become tubercles. These tubercles are surrounded by a little pus, and pierced by a hair, which loosened by the destructive changes going on around it, *will, if pulled, come out, causing scarcely perceptible pain.* This is an eminently contagious form of tinea tricophytina, and is acquired mostly in tonsorial parlors, through the carelessness of barbers. When the tricophyton attacks the nails it produces the disease sometimes called *onychomycosis.*

Tinea kerion from the Greek *kerion* a *honeycomb*, is the name applied by some writers to a form of this variety of tinea, that is simply the result of a more violent action of the tricophyton, in which the hair follicles become specially inflamed and pour out a viscid mucus, resembling the juice of the mistletoe berry.

The *tricophyton*, from *thrix*, a *hair*, and *phuton*, a *plant*, was discovered by Gruby in 1844. It was afterwards more fully described by Bazin, of Paris, in 1854. It has an average diameter of .004 mm. and is composed mostly of spores and mycelia, having but comparatively few granules. The spores are round, almost uniform in size, and look like *fish-roe.* The mycelia appear as slightly greenish tubes more or less filled with granules and jointed. The spores are more abundant on the hairy portions of the body, while the mycelia predominate on the non-hairy regions.

Diagnosis.—The main diseases with which tinea tricophytina is apt to be confounded, are: seborrhœa, eczema, psoriasis, favus, sycosis, and acne.

From seborrhœa, it may be diagnosed by the acute character of the disorder, and by the absence of enlarged follicles and a greasy surface. From the squamous stage of eczema, it may be distinguished by the abrupt marginal form of the eruption, the loosening of the hair, the history of contagion, and the more rapid course. From psoriasis, it may be told, by the history of the case, and the decision of the microscope. From favus, by the absence of the characteristic crusts of the latter, and the different fungus. From sycosis, by the loosened hairs, the characteristic tubercles, and the ever present fungus. And from acne, by its seldom or never appearing on the non-hairy parts of the face, as the cheeks and forehead, which are the favorite seats of acne.

A very easy way to detect the nature of the trouble is, to apply a little chloroform to the suspected part. If fungus is present, it turns whitish-yellow as if sprinkled with sulphur powder, otherwise the appearance is unaltered.

Treatment.—As in tinea favosa so in tinea tricophytina, the cardinal point to be remembered is—*kill the parasite.* This is best done by epilation and the use of parasiticides.

Mercuric bichloride lotion—one (.06) to three grains (.19) to the ounce (32.)—is one of the most useful. Shaving every alternate day, and epilation on the days between, accompanied by a diligent use of the mercuric bichloride lotion, proves a sovereign remedy for the form "barber's itch." Sulphurous acid (absolutely fresh) either as a lotion of fifty per cent. strength, or as a spray, will sometimes do better service on an irritable skin than will the merc. bichl. lotion. Red precipitate ointment, from one-half (2.) to one drachm (4.) to the ounce (32.), may be resorted to if other means fail.

Of internal remedies the following may be mentioned:

SEPIA and *Tellurium* are adapted to the ringworm variety, as occurring on either body or scalp.

For the form, "barber's itch," wrongly termed tinea sycosis, MERC. PRECIP. RUBER, *Kali bich.*, Plantago, Tartar emet., and Cicuta are the main remedies.

Cocculus indicus and the remedies mentioned in the treatment of favus may also be compared.

TINEA VERSICOLOR.

Definition.—Tinea versicolor is characterized by the appearance of fawn-colored patches slightly raised above the level of the skin, accompanied by considerable itching and desquamation.

Synonyms.—Chromophytosis. Pityriasis versicolor.

Symptomatology.—Tinea versicolor is a disease of the superficial cells of the cuticle, caused by the presence of a parasite—the *microsporon furfur*—and has been confusedly termed, by some, pityriasis versicolor. It is the mildest of all the tineæ, and occurs mostly in phthisical patients between the ages of twenty and forty, and attacks women oftener than men. The chest and abdomen are most obnoxious to the disease, which when at all extensive gives to the skin a peculiarly *mapped* appearance.

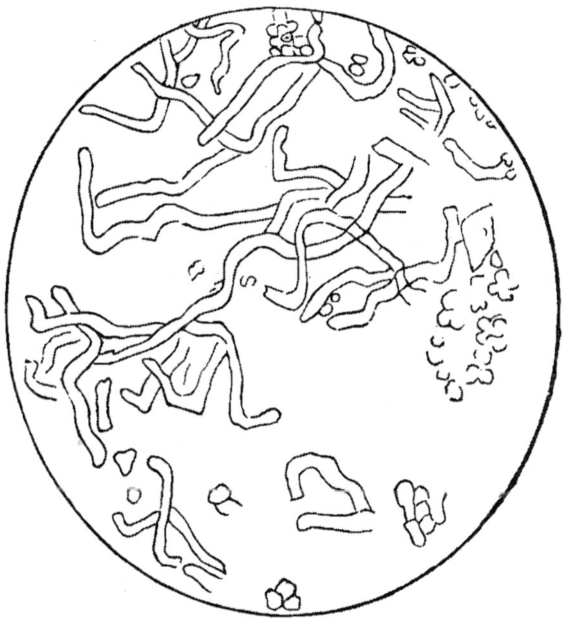

*FIG. 13. MICROSPORON FURFUR.

The *microsporon furfur* (Fig. 13) was discovered by Eichstedt in 1846. Under the microscope its conidia appear of variable size oval or irregularly rounded, and bilinear. They are of a yellowish-gray color,

*From a drawing by Dr. F. R. Day, of this city, taken from a choice specimen found in his private collection.

have an average diameter of .005 mm. and are generally devoid of granules. They manifest a peculiarity in that, *they tend to cluster*, which none of the other conidia do

The mycelia differ but little from those of the tricophyton, only they are shorter, more branched, and are occasionally tipped with *single* spores. They have an average diameter of .0025 mm. The parasite attacks neither hair nor nail. It is the most superficially seated of all the vegetable parasites, having its habitat in the horny layer of the epidermis, and is less tenacious of life than any of the other fungi.

Diagnosis.—The main disease with which tinea versicolor is most liable to be confounded is the erythematous syphilide. The microscope will easily settle this question, even if the syphilitic history of the one does not.

Next to tinea tricophytina it is the most common of the parasitic diseases. It may be found in all classes of society, and tends to run a chronic course. Relapses are frequent, but are more easily managed than in the other varieties of tinea. Its contagious properties are feeble.

Treatment.—The affected parts should be thorougly bathed with soap and water, or an infusion of saponaria bark every day, and the milder parasiticides used. A sulphurous acid (absolutely fresh) or a hypo-sulphite of soda lotion will generally be all that is needed. At times acetic acid baths may be resorted to.

SEPIA and NATRUM ARS., are the principal internal remedies.

TRICHIASIS.

Definition.—Trichiasis is characterized by an abnormal direction of the hair after it leaves the follicle.

Symptomatology.—It affects more commonly the eyelashes, but is occasionally seen on the scalp and eyebrows.

Treatment.—The treatment which is mainly local consists either in pulling out the hairs, which is palliative, or in excising a portion of the palpebral skin if it affects the eyelids, and bringing the edges of the wound together with three or four sutures.

BORAX has been recommended as a useful remedy both internally and locally.

TRICHOCLASIS.

Definition.—Trichoclasis is characterized by brittleness of the hair and the development of little knots along the shaft which look like "nits."

Symptomatology.—It is usually confined to the hair of the beard, and is not contagious.

Treatment.—Shaving off the hair is occasionally necessary. *Natrum mur.* may be given internally, and salt water—Brigg's concentrated sea water—washes used externally.

URTICARIA.

Definition.—Urticaria is an inflammation of the skin, characterized by capriciousness of eruption and the development of reddish or whitish "wheals," attended by tingling and stinging.

Synonyms.—Nettle rash. Hives. Febris urticata.

Symptomatology.—The wheals of this affection vary greatly in size, but are ordinarily of the dimensions of a finger nail—occasionally they attain the size of half an egg (*giant urticaria*)—and are commonly surrounded by an areola. They may be multiform, but are usually roundish or oval. To the touch they may be either soft or hard. When simple or uncomplicated they disappear without leaving any mark or scar. A very annoying, burning, stinging, tingling sensation, likened to the sting of the nettle, is a more or less constant accompaniment, and gives rise to an almost irresistible desire to scratch. And so ephemeral is the disease that "scratch marks" are often all that is left for inspection. The wheals come and go suddenly, are oftentimes excited by simply rubbing the skin, and are prone to change base.

Urticaria occurs at all periods of life, and may appear on any part of the body or mucous membrane; sometimes it attacks the tongue, and the patient may be almost choked.

It usually presents itself as an *acute* disorder, the result of some dietetic error, lasting only a week or two. Occasionally, however, it appears as a *chronic* affection. Sometimes an œdematous condition precedes and accompanies the eruption, and at times an effusion of blood into the wheals, may take place (*U. purpurea.*)

An acute attack is generally ushered in with febrile symptoms, headache, and more or less gastric derangement. The eruption appears suddenly, accompanied by intolerable itching, and the entire surface may be covered in a very short time. After a while, it may be on the removal of the exciting cause, the symptoms begin to subside, and soon all vestiges of the disease have vanished.

Etiology.—Urticaria constitutes about ten per cent of all skin affections. Its causes are many. Organic uterine disease in women, and intestinal irritation in children are not infrequent sources. Acute urticaria may be precipitated by overloading the stomach, or by the excessive use of wine or highly seasoned food. A peculiar idiosyncrasy may cause its appearance after eating crabs, oysters, lobsters, sausage, mushrooms, strawberries, eggs, canned goods, etc. Overdosing with copaiva, cubebs, chloral, turpentine, or valerian will give rise to the rash.

Diagnosis.—Urticaria can hardly be mistaken for any other disease, although it bears some resemblance to dermatitis contusiformis. It, however, wants the lividity, the regular course, the oval shape of the tumors, and the absence of itching of the latter.

Treatment.—All dietetic errors should be corrected, and if an overloaded stomach is the cause, an emetic should be administered. The exciting cause must in all cases be removed as early as possible. Locally, warm vinegar and water lotions may be used to allay the itching and burning. Chloroform and cream mixture—one-half drachm (2.) to the ounce (32.)—will frequently prove serviceable. Favorable mention may also be made of the benzoic acid wash—five (.33) to ten grains (.66) to the ounce (32.) A weak carbolic acid lotion at times acts well. The Turkish bath may help when other means fail.

One of the following internal remedies will generally be indicated:

Allium cepa.—Nettle-rash on the thighs with stitches and burnings. Acute catarrhal symptoms.

Anacardium.—Nettle-rash from emotional causes. Dull pressure as from a plug in various parts. Weakness of memory.

Antimonium crud.—Chronic nettle-rash on the face and joints accompanied by thirst, nausea and thick, white coated tongue. Gastric derangement.

APIS MEL.—Red and inflamed raised patches of hives, with stinging and burning. Aggravated by heat, ameliorated by cold water. Itching and appearance of blotches after scratching. Uterine catarrh. Urine scanty and high colored.

Arsenicum alb.—Wheals of a scarlet color on the face and neck, the size of a half dollar. Intense burning. Itching better from external heat; worse from cold or from scratching.

ASTACUS FLUV.—In chronic cases when other remedies fail. Clay colored stools.

Aurum.—Dirty, yellow blotches on calves and legs with burning. Better in a warm room. Melancholy. In light-haired, scrofulous subjects.

Belladonna.—Bright scarlet red elevated puffy spots, surrounded by a white border. Parts sensitive to the touch. After eating cabbage or sour-krout.

Berberis—Blotches like nettle-rash on the shoulder and right arm, accompanied with burning and stinging. Momentary cold sensation on the parts. Heartburn with soap-sud taste in mouth.

Bryonia.—Nettle-rash with rheumatic pains from atmospheric changes. Symptoms worse from exposure to the heat of the fire.

Caladium.—Nettle-rash on the chest alternating with asthma. Itching and sudden, violent corrosive burning, often on small spots. Worse at night.

Calcarea carb.—Chronic nettle-rash. White elevated hard nettle-rash which disappears in the cold air. Symptoms aggravated by drinking milk. Acidity.

Calcium sulphide.—Chronic nettle-rash on the fingers and hands. Burning and itching of the skin after scratching.

Carbo veg.—Blotches on the calves of the legs, wrists and feet. Burning in various places on the skin. In cachectic individuals, accompanying dyspepsia.

Causticum.—Rash on the thighs just above the knees. Worse during dry, better during wet weather. Chronic nettle-rash.

Cinchona.—Nettle-rash coming out after scratching. Frightful swelling of the face, forearms and hands in the morning. Debility after loss of animal-fluids. Malarial complications.

CIMICIFUGA.—Urticaria from menstrual disorders. Excessive muscular soreness. Brain feels too large for cranium. In nervous hysterical females.

Cina.—White wheals surrounded by erythematous redness, first on the nose, then all over the body. From worms.

Chloral.—Large raised wheals on the arms and legs, coming on suddenly, from a chill. Aggravated by the smallest quantity of wine, beer, or spirits. In grain doses in obstinate cases.

Cocculus.—Hard blotches, surrounded by red areolæ, on the limbs, wrists and back of the fingers. Burning itching as from nettles.

Conium.—Stinging like flea-bites, only one stitch at a time. Evanescent itching.

COPAIVA.—Urticaria at first on the face, especially the forehead, then on the back of the hands, and finally in isolated patches all over the body. Large red blotches, with constipation and fever. Urine scanty and full of sediment. Great restlessness.

Condurango.—Chronic urticaria. Gastric pains, mostly at the cul-de-sac of the stomach.

Dulcamara.—White blotches with red areolæ, on the arms and thighs. Nettle-rash over the whole body without fever. Eruption preceding the menses.

Fagopyrum.—Sore, red blotches inducing scratching, which aggravates. Swelling, the size of a hen's egg, on the neck and shoulder. Dreadful stinging itching.

Graphites.—Red spots like flea-bites all over, especially on the calves of the legs. Itching worse in the evening and at night. Skin dry, never perspires, and is inclined to crack. In females with disposition to delayed menstruation.

Hypericum.—Eruption like nettle-rash on both hands at 4 P. M. Crawling in the hands and feet, they felt fuzzy.

Ignatia.—During chilly stage of intermittent fever. Frequent discharge of much watery urine. In nervous subjects.

KALI CARB.—Urticaria during menstruation. Worse in warm weather. In persons with dry skin, or who are inclined to pulmonary troubles.

Lycopus.—Troublesome urticaria, especially affecting the left forearm and right leg, before eating.

Magnesia carb.—Hard blotches as if from nettle sting, worse during menstruation. Menstrual flow more profuse at night.

Lycopodium.—Itching with nettle-rash eruption on the extremities. Desire to eat, but a small quantity of food fills him up. Inclined to constipation.

Mercurius.—Small flat light-red blotches on the sexual parts, abdomen, chest and inner side of the thighs. Easy perspiration without relief.

Natrum mur.—White blotches on the arms and hands, turning red on scratching. Red blotches over the whole body. Violent itching.

Nux vom.—When accompanied by constipation, vertigo and headache.

Podophyllum.—Intolerable itching of the skin on the body and arms; on scratching it raises up in blotches like hives.

PULSATILLA NIG.—Red, hot spots like nettle-rash. After eating fat pork, fruits or buckwheat.

Pulsatilla nut.—Blotches on the right breast, standing out like measles, with red base, turning white on scratching. Violent itching, worse at night before bed time.

Robinia—Burning itching wherever a part of the face is touched. Itching of skin where rests upon it. Sour stomach.

Sarsaparilla.—Blotches as from nettles. Burning itching with chilliness after abuse of mercury.

Sepia.—Red lentil-sized blotches on the hands. Chronic nettle-rash, especially on the face, arms and thorax. Aggravated by cold. Ameliorated by warmth. After milk and pork.

Solanum oler.—Urticaria febrilis.

Spigelia.—Small elevations like hives on the lower extremities *after scratching*.

Stannum.—Small itching hives below the wrist through the day. Itching aggravated by rubbing. In patients with phthisis.

Sulphur.—Itching hives over the whole body. Aggravated by the warmth of the bed. Chronic cases.

Tartar emetic.—White lumps with red areolæ. Eruption comes and goes. Worse after meat.

Tetradymite —Nettle-rash on face after eating crabs.

Triosteum perf.—Nettle-rash with gastric derangement.

Urtica urens.—Nettle-rash attending or preceding rheumatism. Itching swellings all over the fingers. Aggravated every year at the same time.

Ustilago.—Terrible nightly itching. Menstruation

irregular from ovarian irritation. During the climaxis.

Veratrum alb.—Nettle-rash about the joints only.

Zincum met.—Stinging itching in the skin with nettle-rash eruption after rubbing. Itching rash in hollows of the knees and bends of the elbows. After moderate wine drinking.

VERRUCA.

Definition.—Verruca may be defined as a hypertrophied papilla of the skin, covered with a hypertrophic layer of epidermis.

Synonym.—Wart.

Symptomatology.—Warts may develop as small circumscribed split-pea sized elevations, broad at the base, and of the same color or a little darker than the surrounding skin, or as flat and broad slightly elevated finger nail sized, brownish colored growths. The former develop mostly on the hands in young people, and the latter on the back in elderly persons.

At times they appear as slender, conical, thread-like growths, and are about three millimeters long. These may occur either singly or in groups, and are seen mostly on the neck, face and eyelids.

Digitated broad warts sometimes form on the scalp. They somewhat resemble a crab in appearance, and hence have obtained the vernacular "crab warts."

Venereal warts are pinkish or reddish vascular vegetations, and occur for the most part on the genitals, preferably on the penis and labia. They may also form about the mouth and anus, in the axilla and between the toes. They are apt to grow very rapidlly, and may attain considerable size. They are caused by the contact of irritating fluids, and may be either dry or moist, according to their location. They may occur in connection with gonorrhœa, but are never like the condylomata, a sign of constitutional syphilis.

Treatment.—The smaller warts should be removed by the curved scissors, and the larger and more vascular ones by the curette, ligature or galvano-caustic wire.

Venereal warts need the strictest cleanliness. The dry ones may be treated locally by thuja or mercuric bichloride lotion. The moist ones respond best to dusting with the mercuric chloride.

THUJA has great reputation in removing all kinds of warts.

Moles may be removed by the topical use of the acid nitrate of mercury.

The following are the generally indicated remedies for warts:

Antimonium crud.—Soft smooth warts on the neck, arms and hands.

Berberis.—Warts the size of millet seeds.

Bufo.—Warts on the back of the hands.

CALCAREA CARB.—Small, soft warts.

CINNABAR.—Warts on the prepuce which bleed when touched.

CAUSTICUM.—Warts on the nose and eyebrows. Painful warts.

Dulcamara.—Flat warts.

Lachesis.—Warts on the thumb.

LYCOPODIUM.—Pediculated warts.

Magnesia carb.—May be given two or three grains a day, when other remedies fail.

NATRUM CARB.—Ulcerated warts.

Nitric acid. Soft warts. Warts on the eyelids.

Sepia.—Large, hard warts.

Sulphur.—Hard warts. Warts under the eyes.

THUJA.—Warts on the fingers. Horny, hard warts. It follows well after Calcarea.

WASHERWOMAN'S ITCH.

Definition.—Washerwoman's itch is an inflammation of the skin occurring on the hands in washerwomen. See Eczema.

XANTHOMA.

Definition.—Xanthoma is a connective tissue new growth, characterized by the presence of slightly raised circumscribed "chamois-leather" patches or golden-yellow tubercles.

Synonyms.—Xanthelasma. Vitiligoidea. Fibroma lipomatodes.

Symptomatology.—Its most common seat is the eyelid, near the inner canthus, but it may occur on any part of the body. It never occurs in children, is more common in women than in men, and is frequently associated with jaundice.

The *macular* form appears as yellow rounded, oval, or semi-circular, "chamois-leather" looking patches, unaccompanied by pain. The *tubercular* form consists of rounded, golden-yellow tubercles, varying in size from a pin's-head to a large pea. This variety is found less frequently upon the eyelids than on other parts. In both forms the new growth consists of fibrous tissue containing fat granules, and it is to the latter that the disease owes its color.

Treatment.—Xanthoma can only be cured by removing the patches.

XERODERMA.

Definition.—See Ichthyosis.

ZOSTER.

Definition.—Zoster is an acute disease characterized by the appearance of groups of vesicles upon inflamed bases, along the course of the cutaneous nerves, attended by neuralgic pain.

Synonyms.—Herpes zoster. Zona. Shingles.

Symptomatology.—Like the eruptive fevers, zoster is attended by symptoms preceding the outbreak of the eruption, such as fever and neuralgic pain; the eruption, too, presents definite characters, runs a clearly defined course, and with it the febrile malady disappears. Moreover it rarely attacks the same person twice, and is usually attended by sequela—notably neuralgic pain.

It appears mostly on the chest, along the course of the intercostal nerves, and is generally unilateral. When occurring in the orbital region, it may seriously affect the eye, and is apt to leave behind a severe neuralgia. The eruption is usually preceded by a feeling of prickling, stinging itching of the parts, which lasts from twenty-four to forty-eight hours, and abates on the appearance of the vesicles. The vesicles are at first filled with a clear serum, which soon becomes turbid. They last from eight to ten days, and if not broken, either undergo absorption or dry up and disappear in little brown scales.

Zoster occurs most frequently between the ages of twelve and twenty-four, and attacks males more than females. It is a self limited affection and usually runs its course in from one to two weeks.

Etiology.—Zoster is due to an inflammation of the sympathetic fibres of the ganglia through which the nerves course to the part affected. The eruption involves generally the stratum corneum, the stratum lucidum and the rete, and acts, if the expression is allowed, as the explosion of the nerve disease on the surface. Atmospheric changes and mechanical violence play important parts in its causation.

Diagnosis.—The characters of zoster are usually so well marked, that it can hardly be mistaken for any other affection. From herpes with which it may be confounded, it can be distinguished as follows:

Zoster appears but once in a life time, and is generally unilateral. Herpes is prone to recur and is usually bi-lateral. Zoster is associated with a lesion of some nerve or ganglion, and appears along the course of a nerve or nerves. Herpes follows in the train of catarrhal affections and pneumonia, and is generally confined to the face and genitals. Neuralgic pains precede the eruption of zoster; herpes has only a burning itching. Zoster often leaves cicatrices and a troublesome neuralgia; herpes never does.

Treatment.—The galvanic current from four to eight cells of a battery of ordinary strength, has been found very beneficial if the pain is sharp, when applied from fifteen to twenty minutes daily. The local treatment consists in protecting the vesicles and relieving the neuralgic pain. To this end the parts may be painted with collodion, or dusted with the sub-nitrate of bismuth and starch, equal parts, and a protective bandage applied. Chaulmoogra oil will oftentimes prove a very beneficial application. Cantharis lotion has been highly recommended, and will at times be of service.

RHUS TOX., is the principal internal remedy.

Others may be indicated as follows:

Aconite.—In the earlier stages, when the neuralgic pain is accompanied by febrile symptoms.

Apis.—Burning and stinging pains with swelling. Large vesicles, sometimes confluent. Better from cold applications.

ARSENICUM ALB.—Confluent eruption with *intense burning* of the blisters. Worse after midnight, and from cold applications. Neuralgia. In debilitated constitutions.

Cantharis.—Large blisters, burning when touched. Smarting and stinging. Mostly on the right side. Worse in the open air.

CISTUS.—Zoster on the back. Neuralgic symptoms. In scrofulous subjects.

COMOCLADIA.—Zoster on the legs. Rheumatic pains aggravated by rest; relieved by motion.

DULCAMARA.—Zoster after taking cold from damp air. Moist, suppurating eruption. Glandular swellings in neighborhood of eruption. Eruption precedes the menses.

GRAPHITES.—Zoster on the left side. Large blisters from the spine to the umbilicus, burning when touched. Worse indoors. Better in the open air. Dry skin, tendency to ulceration. In blonde individuals inclined to obesity.

Iris versicolor.—Zoster especially on the right side. Following gastric derangement. Pain in the liver. Neuralgic pains.

KALMIA LAT.—Facial neuralgia remaining after zoster. Worse at night. Palpitation of the heart. Rheumatic pains.

Lachesis.—Zoster during spring and fall. The vesicles turn dark and are very painful. All symptoms are worse after sleep.

MERCURIUS.—Zoster on the right side, extending across the abdomen. Worse at night, from the warmth of the bed. Tendency to suppuration. Easy perspiration without relief.

MEZEREUM.—Zoster in old people. Constant chilliness. Neuralgic pains. Worse at 9 P. M. Burning, changing location after scratching. In scrofulous persons.

Ranunculus bulb.—Zoster aggravated by change of temperature. Neuralgic sequels. In rheumatic subjects.

Rhus tox.—Burning and stinging pains aggravated by scratching. Small burning vesicles with redness of the skin. Confluent vesicles. Worse in cold weather. Rheumatic pains during rest. Sleeplessness with restless tossing about. Zoster brought on by getting wet, while over-heated.

Sempervivium tect.—In obstinate cases. May be used internally and locally.

Thuja.—Zoster with eruption only on covered parts. Better from gentle rubbing. In individuals of lymphatic temperament.

Zincum.—Neuralgia following zoster. Pains relieved by touching the parts. Worse after dinner and towards evening.

Zincum phos.—When other remedies fail. Following brain-fag in literary persons.

PART III.—A CHART OF CHARACTERISTICS

With Diagnostic, Therapeutic, Dietetic, and Hygienic Hints.

CLASS.	DISEASES.	DEFINITIONS AND DIAGNOSTIC FEATURES.	THERAPEUTIC, DIETETIC AND HYGIENIC HINTS.
I. DISORDERS OF THE GLANDS.	ANIDROSIS.	Functional disease of the perspiratory apparatus. Characterized by *insufficient sweat*. May be either congenital or acquired.	Æthusa, Plumbum, etc. Turkish baths. Free use of water internally and externally.
	BROMIDROSIS. (Osmidrosis.)	Functional disorder of sweat glands. Characterized by *offensive sweat*. Most in axillæ and feet. General or local.	Conium mac, (*acrid.*) Petroleum, (*axillæ*). Silicea, (*feet*). Staphysagria, (*rotten*). Zincum, (*profuse*), etc. Alum or Carbolic acid lotion and Diachylon plaster dressings. Strictest cleanliness.
	CHROMIDROSIS.	Functional disorder of sweat glands. Characterized by *colored perspiration*. Fitful secretion. In hypochondriacs and unmarried women with uterine disorders.	Nux Vomica.
	COMEDO. (Grub.)	Disorder of sebaceous glands Characterized by small black-topped, sebaceous points. Chin, forehead and cheeks. Young people. Face looks as if sprinkled with gunpowder.	Baryta carb. Selenium, Sumbul, etc. Remove "grubs" with comedo extractor. Sulphur lotion. Matrimony. Exclude fatty food.

I. DISORDERS OF THE GLANDS.			
	Sebaceous Cyst. (Wen.)	A white, round or oval tumor, of variable size, composed of sebaceous matter enclosed in a sac. Single or multiple. Painless. Scalp, face and neck.	Potassium iodide. Baryta or Bromine. Excision.
	Hyperidrosis.	Functional disorder of sweat glands. Characterized by *excessive sweat*. General or local. Symmetrical or unilateral. Local. Most on head. hands. feet and genitals. Flat-footed people.	Baptisia. Boletus. Calc. carb. Jaborandi. Lactic acid. Selenium, etc. Use as little water as possible.
	Miliaria. (Prickly heat.)	Disordered action of the sweat glands. Characterized by numerous pin-head sized reddened papules or vesico-papules attended with heat and tingling. Trunk usual seat. May appear on neck, face and arms. More in summer. Apt to relapse.	Bryonia. Arsenicum alb. Raphanus, etc. Carbolated bran baths. followed by dusting with sub-nitrate of bismuth and starch, or lycopodium powder. Cast off superfluous clothing.
	Milium. (Skin-stones.)	Disorder of sebaceous glands. Characterized by white, roundish sebaceous points beneath the epidermis. size from millet-seed to a split-pea. Eyelids and forehead. More common in women than in men.	Calcium iodide and Staphysagria, and Tabacum. Remove by knife. Use Saponaria bark wash.

I. DISORDERS OF THE GLANDS.			
	MOLLUSCUM SEBACEUM.	Disease of sebaceous glands. Characterized by roundish, pea-sized tumors, umbilicated in the center and of a pinkish white color. Face mostly. In children. May be semi-epidemic. Tumors contain cheesy matter.	Silicea and Teucrium. Calc. ars. Bromine, etc. In early stage, Acid nitrate of Mercury, locally. If tumors are large use the knife.
	SEBORRHŒA. (Sebaceous flux.)	Functional disorder of sebaceous glands. Characterized by *excessive secretion of sebum.* On face and scalp. More in women than in men. Appears in the light complexioned, as an *oily coating;* and in the dark complexioned, as dirty white or yellow flat scales, (dandruff).	Bufo. Bryonia. Calc. carb. Kali carb. Natrum. Plumbum. Raphanus, etc. Locally, in *mild cases.* Saponaria bark wash. Glyceral tannin, or tannin and rice powder, (*face*). In *chronic cases.* Sapo viridis. Merc. cor. lotion, or Red precipitate oint. Keep system in healthy state.
	SUDAMINA.	Disorder of sweat glands, Characterized by pin-head sized vesicles, formed by the collection of sweat between the layers of epidermis. In summer and in acute diseases. Sign of general debility.	Bryonia, Ammonium mur., and Urtica urens. Look after the general health.

II. INFLAMMATIONS.			
	ACNE. (Stone-pock.)	Disease of the sebaceous glands. Caused by retention of sebum. Characterized by papules, tubercles and pustules. Pin-head or pea-sized elevations around glandular orifices. On face and back. At puberty. From gastric derangement, functional derangement of sexual system. Tar, etc.	Ant. crud. Bell. Chel. maj. Granatum. Kali. bich. Kali. bromat. Potass. iod. Nit. acid. Nux. jug. Ledum. Phos. acid. Sulphur. Sumbul, etc. Extract comedos. Stimulating lotions in mild forms. Soothing applications in severe cases. Rumex lotion. Merc. corr. Merc. jodat, and Bi-jodat (*indurated*). Light diet. Sea-salt baths.
	ANTHRAX. (Carbuncle.)	Phlegmonous inflammation, characterized by necrosis of the cellular tissue, with suppuration and the discharge of the necrosed masses, called *cores*, with pus, through corresponding sieve-like openings. Circumscribed. Commences with burning pains. Size from a fifty-cent piece to a saucer. On nape of neck, shoulders, forehead and buttocks. More in winter. May be epidemic.	Anthracinum. Ars. alb. Arctium lappa. Nit. acid. Lachesis. Phytolacca. Silicea, etc. Locally: Ice-bags in early stages. Later: hot flaxseed meal poultices. Nourishing diet. Brandy and egg, etc.
	DERMATITIS CONTUSIFORMIS. (Erythema nodosum.)	Characterized by oval or round purplish nodules, varying in size from a hickory nut to a fist. Febrile disturbance. Nodules form suddenly. Never suppurate. Fade away like bruises. Anterior surface of leg. Young persons, especially females. Relapses.	Rhus venenat. Arnica. Ptelea trif., etc. Locally: Arnica or Hamamelis. Horizontal posture.

II. INFLAMMATIONS.	DERMATITIS EXFOLIATIVA. (Pityriasis rubra.)	Characterized by highly reddened skin, and abundant exfoliation of epidermis in *large white flakes*. Whole surface. Handfuls of flakes shed. Adult life. Involves papillary layer. Due to disturbance of trophic nerves.	Ars. alb. Ars. jodat. Kali ars. Piper methyst., etc. Bran baths or decoction of walnut leaves, followed by oily inunctions. Tarry preparations.
	DYSIDROSIS.	Disease of sweat structures of hands and feet. Characterized by redness and swelling of the parts, with distension of the sweat ducts in the shape of *sago-like points*, and the development of bullæ. In summer. The nervously debilitated. Attacks symmetrically the fingers, palms and soles.	Clematis and Natrum sulph. Alkaline starch baths. Carron oil.
	ECTHYMA.	Characterized by large, isolated, painful pustules, situated upon hard and inflamed bases, and followed by dark brown crusts. Slight fever. Superficial lesion. Develops rapidly. On neck, shoulders and back.	Ars. alb. Merc. Tart. emet., etc. Weak, White Precipitate oint. Carbolic acid wash. Generous diet.

II. INFLAMMATIONS.	ECZEMA. (Salt-rheum.) (Grocer's itch.) (Washerwoman's itch.)	Simple inflammation of the skin, characterized by an erythematous, papular, vesicular or pustular eruption with burning and itching. Discharge stiffens linen. Acute or chronic. Light florid complexioned individuals. Head in infancy. Trunk and genitals in adult life. Itching. Greenish yellow crusts. Due to faulty innervation.	Ars. alb. Bovista, Calc. carb. Croton tig. Graph. Nux. jug. Oleander. Rhus. Sarsap. Sulphur, etc. Locally—Early; Bran washes, emollient poultices, etc. Later: Zinc and starch, Lycopodium or Glyceral tannin. For itching: Dioscorea, Carbolic acid or Hydrocyanic acid, lotions or Grindel. cerate (*acute cases*); pyroligneous oil of Juniper (*in non-inflammatory cases*). Benz. oxide of Zinc oint. or Oleate of Litharge. White or red precipitate oint. Chrysophanic cerate (*squamous stage*). Sapo viridis (*chronic.*) Oil of white birch.
	ERYTHEMA.	Characterized by macules, papules or tubercles, attended by more or less itching and burning. Redness disappears under pressure leaves a yellow spot, which becomes red again. In children and young people. On back of hands and feet, arms, legs and forehead. Spring and fall. Known by its superficial protean character, and general distribution.	Aconite. Ars. iodat. Bell. Chel. maj. Chloral hydrate. Lactic acid. Mezereum. Nux. vom. Ustilago, etc. Carbolic acid. Grindelia or Verat. vir., lotion. Oxide of Zinc or Lycopodium powder.

II. INFLAMMATIONS.	FURUNCLE. (Boil.)	Circumscribed inflammation of the skin and connective tissue, varying in size from a small pea to a hickory nut, having an indurated and inflamed base, and terminating in suppuration and the formation of a "*core.*" On face, back and gluteal region. Dependent on disordered blood states or depraved conditions of system.	Ant. crud. Bell. Bellis perennis. Calc. carb. Calc. mur. Calc. sulph. Gels. Nitric acid. Nux. jug. Phos. acid. Rhus rad., etc. Muriate of Lime lotion. Flax-seed or tomato poultices. Gelsemium or Lappa cerate. Well hygiened. Good wholesome diet.
	HERPES. (Fever blister.)	Acute. Characterized by *groups of vesicles*, having reddened slightly inflamed bases, and situated *on face and genitals.* Febrile symptoms. Heat, redness and swelling. Vesicles larger than in eczema, but smaller than in zoster. Excited by cold. May be symptomatic.	Aconite. Ars. alb. Bufo. Calcium sulph. Kali bich. Merc. sol. Natrum mur. Sarsaparilla, etc. Camphorated cream or cologne water, locally.
	HYDROA.	Characterized by isolated vesicles which tend to recur. Starts as little papules. Itching. Symmetrical. On face, exterior surfaces of limbs and genitals. Two or three weeks duration.	Potass. iod. Kreasote. Magnesia carb., etc. Salzburg springs.

II. INFLAMMATIONS.	HYDRO-ADENITIS.	Inflammation of perspiratory follicles and adjacent connective tissue, terminating in suppuration. Bright red, pea-sized swellings. Suppurate in a few days. In axillæ, around nipple and on perineum. Has no core.	Phos. acid, (*axillæ*). Phosphorus, (*nipple*). Nit. acid, (*perineum*). Gels., or Lappa lotion. Tomato poultices. Hot fomentations.
	IMPETIGO CONTAGIOSA.	Characterized by one or more discrete vesicles or vesico-pustules, generally umbilicated, varying in size from a split pea to a hazel-nut, and followed by flat, straw-colored, usually fungoid crusts. Acute. Contagious. Febrile symptoms. Vesicles grow rapidly and have red areolæ. Crusts, straw-colored, flat, and looks as if stuck on. Runs its course in one or two weeks. Most on forehead and cheeks. May extend to mucous membrane. Wake of vaccination.	Ant. crud. Aconite. Euphorbium. Tart. emet. Kali bich. Silicea, etc. Soothing applications. White precipitate ointment. Well nourished.

II. INFLAMMATIONS	INTERTRIGO.	A hyperæmic affection. Characterized by heat, redness and an abraded surface, with maceration of epidermis. From contact of two cutaneous surfaces. In fat persons and in infants.	Calc. carb. Cham. Graph. Petroleum. Nux. jug., etc. Wash with soap and water. Dust with Lycopodium or Oxide of Zinc, and rice powder.
	LICHEN PLANUS.	Characterized by dull, red, flat topped, angular based, pinhead sized, glazed papules. Chronic. Runs a papular course. Itching. Symmetrical. Leave melasmic stains. Front of forearms and wrists, thighs, abdomen and leg below the knee. More in women. Disturbance of the trophic nerves of hair papillæ, with hyperæmia and new tissue formation.	Ant. crud. Ars. alb. Kali bich. Nux. jug., etc. Carbolic acid, Grindelia or Hydrocyanic acid dil. wash. Pyroligneous oil of Juniper. Liberally fed and well hygiened.

II. INFLAMMATIONS.	LICHEN SIMPLEX.	Characterized by round, solid millet-seed, sized, flesh-colored, or reddish papules. Itching. Distinctly papular course. Outer aspects of forearm, neck and thigh.	Anatherium. Ant. crud. Ars. alb. Bell. Caladium. Kreasote. Ledum. Nux. jug. Plantago maj. Rumex. Sulphur, etc. Locally: Cyanide of Potasium, Borax, or Merc. corr., wash. White precipitate or Iodide of Sulphur oint. Glyceral tannin.
	PEMPHIGUS.	Characterized by bullæ, in groups of three or four, and varying in size from a pea to a hickory nut. Mostly chronic. *P. Vulgaris* on limbs and ankles. Blisters round or oval. *Successive crops. P. Foliaceus* starts as single flaccid bulla on sternum. Spreads over whole surface. Dry up and form *yellow parchment-like flakes.*	Rhus tox., (*acute*). Ars. alb., (*chronic*). Thuja, (*foliaceus*). Causticum. Phos. acid. Ran. bulb., etc. Bran, starch, gelatine or the continuous bath. Animal diet. Fresh air and plenty of exercise.

II. INFLAMMATIONS.			
	PERNIO. (Chilblain.)	Acute. Secondary effect of cold. Appears mostly on hands and feet. Ulcers may form. A winter disease mostly.	Agaricus. Ars. alb. Canth. Citrus vulg. Petroleum. Urtica dioica. Verat. vir., etc. Locally: Decoction of marshmallows, (*inflamed*). Tamus com. tinct., (*unbroken*). Diachylon plaster, Oxide of Zinc oint. or Glycercole of Calendula, (*broken*). Resin oint., (*ulcers*). Tinct. of Benzoin as preventive.
	PITYRIASIS. (Branny tetter.)	Characterized by fine, dry, bran-like scales, seated on slightly reddened, non-infiltrated surface. Slight itching. On scalp, face and trunk. Seated in deep layers of epidermis, and consists in excessive cell proliferation.	Ars. alb. Fluoric acid. Kali ars., etc. Locally: Infusion of Saponaria bark, or Glycerole of Borax.
	PRAIRIE ITCH.	Acute. Appears in new districts. May be epidemic. Headache, malaise. Slight fever. Vesicles, pin-head or mustard-seed sized. *Intense itching.* "*Scratch marks.*" Large blackish scales. Boils. On neck, shoulders, back and outer surface of limbs.	Rumex crisp. Rhus. tox. Ledum, etc. Locally: Diluted lye of wood ashes. Hepar sulph. Kali lotion.

II. INFLAMMATIONS.	PRURIGO.	Characterized by small papules of same color as skin, accompanied by intense itching. Skin dry, rough, harsh and thickened. "Scratch marks." Exterior surfaces of lower extremities mostly. Starts before puberty. Worse in winter. May continue through life. Due to chronic changes in the papillary layer.	Sulphur. Ars. alb. Ambra. Dioscorea. Dolichos prur. Oleander. Nitric acid, etc. Carbolic acid or Mezereum lotion. Tar or Sulphur baths. Nutritious diet.
	PSORIASIS. (Dry Tetter.)	Constitutional disease. Characterized by reddish thickened patches, covered with whitish or yellowish white, mother-of-pearl colored scales. Develops rapidly. Elbows and knees mostly. Apt to be symmetrical. Scales are imbricated. Of malarial or traumatic origin. Due to perversion of cell life of the rete.	Ars. alb. Ars. jod. Merc. sol. Muriatic acid. Phos. Sul, etc. Locally: Saponaria bark, or bran baths. Inunctions with Cod-liver or Chaulmoogra oil. Iodide of Sulphur or Chrysophanic cerate. Oil of white birch. Biniodide of Mercury or white precipitate oint. Green soap treatment. Generous diet. Cod-liver oil.

II. INFLAMMATIONS.	STROPHULUS. (Red-gum). (Tooth-rash).	Characterized by small, red or white papules, varying in size from a pin's head to a millet seed. On face, neck and arms, mostly. Two forms. Due to congestion about the mouths of sweat follicles.	Chamomilla. Calcarea carb. Spiranthes. Borax. Ledum. Apis. Cicuta. Sumbul, etc.
	URTICARIA. (Nettle-rash). (Hives).	Characterized by sudden development of *wheals*, of a whitish or reddish color, attended by itching and burning. Wheals are usually round or oval, and finger-nail sized. Come and go suddenly. "Scratch-marks." May be ushered in by febrile symptoms. Caused by dietetic errors, organic uterine disease, and intestinal irritation.	Apis mel. Berberis. Calcarea carbonica. Cimicifuga. Chloral hydrate. Cina. Copaiva. Condurango. Ignatia. Kali carb. Natrum. Puls. nig. Robinia. Sulphur, Ustilago, etc. Locally: Vinegar and water, or Chloroform and cream. Benzoic acid or Carbolic acid lotion. Turkish baths. Remove exciting cause.

II. INFLAMMATIONS.	ZOSTER. (Shingles).	Characterized by groups of split-pea sized vesicles, seated along the course of nerves, and attended by neuralgic pain. Resembles eruptive fevers. Between ages of 12 and 24. Runs course in 2 or 3 weeks. *Unilateral.* Often leaves cicatrices. Neuralgia, a sequel. Due to inflammation of sympathetic fibres of ganglia.	Rhus toxicodendron. Comocladia. Graphites. Dulcamara Kalmia. Mercurius. Mezereum. Zincum met. Zincum phos., etc. Galvanic current. Locally: Collodion, or Subnitrate of Bismuth and starch, dusting powder. Chaulmoogra oil, or Cantharis lotion.
III. HÆMORRHAGES.	PURPURA.	Characterized by an effusion of red blood globules into the cutis, usually unattended by constitutional disturbance. Spots first bright red, then purple, and change color like a bruise. On legs, mostly. Usually symmetrical. More in aged. Occur in crops. Run a course of 8 or 10 days. May be hæmorrhage from mucous membrane (*land-scurvy*). There is then constitutional disturbance.	Ars. alb. (*simple*). Sulphuric acid (*hæmorrhagic*). Baptisia. Bryonia. Chloral hydrate. Rhus tox. Phos. Veratrum vir., etc. Hamamelis, locally. Malt foods. Outdoor exercise.

IV. HYPERTROPHIES.	OF PIGMENT.	CHLOASMA. (Liver spots).	A coloration of the skin, characterized by round or oval, nickel-sized or larger, yellowish or brownish patches. On face mostly. More in women than in men.	Argent nit. Guaræa. Laurocerasus. Petroleum. Sepia, etc. Locally: Merc. cor. lotion, or Muriate of Lime solution.
		LENTIGO. (Freckle).	A discoloration of skin, due to deposit of pigment in the rete mucosum, is characterized by round, yellowish, split-pea sized spots. On cheeks and back of hands. Light-complexioned, red-haired people.	Kali carb. Sepia. Sulphur, etc. Merc. cor. lotion.
	OF EPID. AND PAP. LAYERS.	CALLOSITAS. (Callosity).	Yellowish or whitish, nickel-sized, horny, elevated patches. On hands and feet. Caused by friction. More in men.	Graphites (*hands*). Silicea (*feet*).
		CLAVUS. (Corn).	A small, usually split-pea sized, flat, horny formation, more or less deeply seated, and painful on pressure. May be hard or soft.	Ant. crud. (*hard corns*). Sulph. (*soft corns*). Corn plasters (*protection*). Verat. vir. lotion (*if inflamed*), etc. Wear easy fitting boots.

IV. HYPETROPHIES.	OF EPIDERMAL AND PAPILLARY LAYERS.	ICHTHYOSIS. (Fish-skin Disease.)	A congenital chronic disease, characterized by dryness and roughness. Mildest form in children (Xeroderma). Furfuraceous scales. In severer cases, papillæ enlarged, lozenge-shaped scales, lines and fissures. In worst cases, scales are yellowish or greenish. They never overlap. May be heaped up into projections. Whole surface more or less involved.	Ars. iodat. Aurum. Clematis. Kali hyd. Phos. Plumbum. Thuja, etc. Turkish baths, and anointing with either Olive. Chaulmoogra, or Cod-liver oil. Infusion of Saponaria bark. Sapo viridis treatment. Generous diet. Cod liver oil.
		VERRUCA. (Wart.)	An enlarged papilla, variable as to size and shape, covered with an hypertrophic layer of epidermis. Split-pea sized, skin-colored on the hands. Finger-nail sized and brownish on back. Conical thread-like growths on neck, face, and eyelids. Digitated warts on scalp. Venereal warts are pinkish, or reddish vascular vegetations.	Calc. carb. Cinnabar. Caust. Lycop. Natrum. Thuja, etc. Remove smaller warts by scissors, and larger ones by ligature or galvano-caustic wire. For dry ones use Thuja, locally. For moist ones, dust with Proto-Chloride of Mercury.

IV. HYPERTROPHIES.	OF CONNECTIVE TISSUE.	ELEPHANTIASIS. (Elephant leg.)	Chronic disease. Characterized by great hypertrophy of skin, and subcutaneous connective tissue, usually confined to the lower limbs and genitals. Ushered in by chill, followed by febrile symptoms. Swelling of leg, painfully distended lymphatics. Due to the *filaria sanguinis*. In malarial districts and tropical climates.	Myristica. Hydrocotyle. Anacardium. Elæis, etc. Esmarch's bandage. Compression of main artery. Excision of sciatic nerve. Hamamelis or Chaulmoogra oil, dressings. Milk diet. Change of climate.
		FRAMBŒSIA. (Yaws.)	An endemic contagious disease. Characterized by variously-sized reddish papules, tubercles and tumors, in all stages of development. Start as pin-head-sized points. First resemble a *currant*, then a *raspberry*, and lastly a *cherry*. Rarely occurs twice. Mostly on face and genitals. Endemic in West Indies, etc.	The Iodides of Mercury and Potassium. Jatropha lotion.

IV. HYPERTROPHIES.	OF CONNECTIVE TISSUE.	ROSACEA. (Copper-nose.) (Wine-nose.)	A chronic disease. Affects more particularly the nose, cheeks and forehead, results from dilatation of the blood-vessels, with increased growth of connective tissue, and is characterized by redness, and a tendency to the development of tubercles and pustules. Three stages: First, passive hyperæmia, nose cold. Second, minute bloodvessels appear. Third, vessels enlarge, skin becomes thickened, papules and tubercles develop. Disease of middle life.	Arsen. bromide. Agaricus. Bromine. Carbo an. Nux. vom. Petroleum. Rhus rad. etc. Sulphur or Merc. corr. lotions (*first stage*). Incision of vessels. Faradic current (*second stage*.) Excision of redundant tissue, etc.
		SCLERODERMA. (Hide-bound disease.)	A chronic affection. Characterized by hardness and inelasticity of integument. Skin has a yellowish-brown waxy appearance. Apt to be symmetrical. Due to stagnation of lymph in the lymph spaces.	Ant. crud. Alumina. Berberis. Elæis. Rhus tox., etc. Galvanism.

IV. HYPERTROPHIES.	OF CONNECTIVE TISSUE.	SCLERIASIS.	An induration of cellular tissue, in new-born children. May be congenital or appear during early months of infant life. Stearine-like deposit in the sub cutaneous tissues. Usually fatal.	Elæis guineensis.
	OF NAIL.	ONYCHOGRYPHOSIS.	Characterized by twisted bent nails, which are thickened, and of a yellowish or brownish color. Mostly nails of toes and fingers. Attacks old people.	Graphites and Silicea.

IV. HYPERTROPHIES.	OF CUTIS.	DERMATOLYSIS.	A hypertrophy of the skin assuming the form of pendulous purse-like folds. Seldom appears before puberty. Runs a chronic course.	Bromide of Ammonium. Large folds may be ligatured or excised.
V. ATROPHIES.	OF PIGMENT.	LEUCODERMA. (Acquired Piebald Skin.)	Characterized by localized loss of pigment. Patches round or oval, of milk white color. Usually on face, hands, and genitals. Adult life. Prognosis unfavorable.	Sulphide of Arsenicum. Natrum. Nitric acid. Phosphide of Zinc, etc. Galvanism. Locally: Acetic acid for pigmentation around the patch.
	OF CONNECTIVE TISSUE.	MORPHŒA.	Characterized by roundish, dirty alabaster-looking patches, circumscribed by lilac-tinted borders, and varying in diameter from half an inch to two inches. Course of left supra-orbital nerve most frequent seat. Runs slow course. May recover spontaneously.	Phosphorus. Constant galvanic current. Well fed. Cod Liver or Chaulmoogra oil.

V. ATROPHIES.	OF NAIL.	ATROPHY OF THE NAIL.	May be either congenital or acquired, and is characterized by deficient growths of nail substance. Nails are brittle and look as if worm-eaten. Have a leaden hue.	**Silicea.**
	OF CUTIS.	LINEAR ATROPHY.	Characterized by white or claret colored, depressed, scar-like streaks or spots. Streaks are one or two lines broad by several inches long. Spots vary from pin's head to a pea in size. Mostly on the thighs. Due to cessation of trophic nerve influence in localized areas.	Cocculus (*claret spots*). Sulphur or Graphites (*white spots*). Sabadilla (*streaks*). Cod-liver oil.

VI. NEW GROWTHS.	OF CONNECTIVE TISSUE.			
		FIBROMA. (Polypus of the Skin.)	Characterized by sessile or pedunculated outgrowths, from the connective tissue, generally club-shaped, and varying in size from a pea to a large pear. Painless. Small ones are soft. The large ones are elastic and fibrous. Large ones may ulcerate.	Cal. ars. Lycop, etc. Remove large tumors by knife elastic ligature or galvano — caustic. Smaller ones disappear under Acid nitrate of Mercury, locally.
		KELOID.	Characterized by one or more flattish smooth-surfaced tumors, usually upon the site of cicatrices. Tumor is made up of a body having numerous prolongations or claws. Size of five-cent piece or larger. Mostly on sternum mammæ. Adult life. Negroes. Spontaneous evolution may take place.	Fluoric acid. Graph. Nit. acid. Sabina, etc. Galvanism.
		XANTHOMA.	Characterized by variously sized golden-yellow, non-indurated macules or tubercles. On eyelid and inner canthus. Women mostly. "Chamois-leather" patches. Golden-yellow tubercles. Consists of fibrous tissue containing fat granules.	Removal of the patch.

VI. NEW GROWTHS.	OF BLOOD-VESSELS.	NÆVUS. (Port-wine stain.) (Mother's-mark.)	A *congenital formation* seated in the skin and subcutaneous tissue. May be either pigmentary or vascular. *Pigmentary* are dark colored sharply defined spots. When covered with hair they are called " mouse marks." *Vascular* nævi may be arterial or venous. Redish or purplish color.	Carbo veg. (*pigmentary*). Thuja (*vascular*). Condurango, Calcarea carb., etc. Locally: for pigmentary. Collodion and Merc. cor. paint. For vascular, Electrolysis or the subcutaneous ligature.
		TELANGIECTASIS.	Characterized by circumscribed vascular cutaneous growths, *appearing* for the most part *during adult life*. Bright red pin-head or split pea sized. On face and neck. may terminate spontaneously, or remain through life.	Same treatment as nævus. Condurago.

VI. NEW GROWTHS.	OF GRANULATION TISSUE.	EPITHELIOMA. (Epithelial cancer.)	An affection of middle life. May start either as a flat infiltration, a wart or other growth. Earliest sign a simple crack, or hard pale dusky lump which sooner or later fissures. Typical ulcer is roundish, split-pea size or larger, has hard sharply defined edges, and secretes a scanty yellow viscid fluid. This form is met with in smokers. Selects as seat the lower lip. On the scrotum it is *chimney sweeper's cancer*. On the upper part of face, *rodent ulcers*. *Second form* commences as papules, which grow, and later tend to form reddish or purplish, walnut-sized aggregations. Sharp pains. Ulcerate. Ulcers have hard, everted, indurated and undermined edges, secrete an offensive pale yellow viscid fluid, and bleed easily. Patient may eventually die from exhaustion. Attacks mucous membrane of cheeks preferably. *Third form*, may develop as wart-like growths or cauliflower excresences. Split-pea or hazel-nut sized. Runs course of second form mostly. E. Originates in the endothelium of the lymphatics.	Thuja. Ars. alb. Condurango, and Red-clover. blossom tea. Locally: Arsenical mucilage. The knife, or the galvano caustic.

VI. NEW GROWTHS.	OF GRANULATION TISSUE.	LEPROSY.	A constitutional disease. Characterized by formation of a new growth, resembling granulation tissue, usually resulting in the destruction of the parts, with anæsthesia and great deformity. Endemic in some countries. Warm climates. Macular. Tubercular. Anæsthetic. Gradual decline in health. *Macular:* faint brownish patches or bullæ followed by scars and pigmentation, patches are dirty-grey color in center, and brownish at periphery. Hyperæsthesia at first, then *anæsthesia.* On trunk and extensor surfaces of extremities. *Tubercular:* Dull brownish-red tubercles varying in size from a pea to a plum. Mostly on face. *Leonine* expression. Ulceration.	Hydrocotyle. Piper methysticum. Calotropis gig. Graph. Sepia. Hura brazil. Guano. Cuprum, etc. Locally: Warm baths and Gurjun oil inunctions. Generous diet. Cod liver or Chaulmoogra oil. Segregation of the lepers.
		LUPUS ERYTHEMATOSUS. (Erythematous scrofulide. (Butterfly lupus.)	Characterized by one or more usually roundish or oval, variably-sized, reddish patches, covered with fine, thin whitish or grayish fatty adherent scales. Pin-head sized pale red spots on cheeks and nose. Centers marked by greenish comedo-points. Covered with adherent fatty scales. Follicles distended and patulous. Seldom before the 20th year. Extend at periphery.	Iodine. Guaraca. Hydrocotyle. Cistus. Apis, etc. Locally: Saponaria bark or Sulphur baths. Oil of white birch. Curette. Good diet. Fresh air and frequent bathing.

VI. NEW GROWTHS.	OF GRANULATION TISSUE.	Disease	Description	Treatment
		LUPUS VULGARIS. (Tubercular scrofulide.) (Wolf.)	A disease of the derma, characterized by variously-shaped, pea-sized or larger, yellowish or reddish elevations, which usually terminate in ulceration and cicatrization. Begins as yellow or red solid points, which enlarge to form tubercles. May terminate by insensible absorption or ulceration. Puberty. Face and extremities. Crusts after ulceration, are brownish-red and scanty. Cicatrices are shrunken and yellowish.	Ars. alb. Cistus. Graph. Guaraca. Hydrocotyle. Staphysagra, etc. Locally: Early stage, Bin-iodide of Mercury oint. Later, Irido-platinum needle dipped in fused Nitrate. Arsenical mucilage. Cosme's paste. Pyrogallic oint. Curette. Nutritious diet. Fresh air. Outdoor exercise.
		RHINO-SCLEROMA.	Characterized by irregularly-shaped, sharp bordered, flat swellings, of a normal or dark reddish-brown color, occurring mostly on nose and upper lip. Unattended by pain, but sensitive to pressure.	Calcarea phos. Guaraca. Rhus rad., etc. Removed by using the irido-platinum points and Squibb's fused Nitrate.

VI. NEW GROWTHS.	OF GRANULATION TISSUE.	SARCOMA CUTIS.	Consists of brownish-red or bluish-red, variously-sized tubercles or nodules, attended by a diffused thickening of the skin. A rare and malignant disease. Occurs mostly in adult life. Usually terminates fatally.	Calc. phos. Silicea. Condurango. Nitric acid, etc.
		SCROFULODERMA.	A strumous disease of the skin, commencing as indolent, painless, livid tubercles, that slowly soften and give place to unhealthy ulcers, with free incrustation. Mostly on neck and beneath the lower jaw. Occasionally on thorax, in axillæ and on groins.	Calcium sulphide. Calcium iodide. Theridion. Scrofularia, etc. Locally: Iodide of starch paste to ulcers. Generous diet. Out-door exercise. Fresh air. Cod-liver oil.
		SYPHILIDES. (Syphilis of the Skin.)	Manifestations of general syphilis on the skin. May be secondary or tertiary. Have a history of syphilitic inoculation. Are of a reddish yellow-brown color. Are polymorphous. Are devoid of pain and itching. Crusts are thick, greenish black. Ulcers are of an ash-gray color, often serpiginous or *horse-shoe* shaped. Diffused eruptions, generally symmetrical, later irregularly distributed. Scales are thin and occur in small circular spots. Are non-inflammatory and tend to recur.	

VI. NEW GROWTHS.	OF GRANULATION TISSUE.	SYPHILIDES.			
			Papular.	Flat split-pea sized or larger, slightly raised patches. Earliest manifestation. No itching. May last for months, significant signs of syphilis attend it.	Merc. jodat. Merc. corr. Locally: White precipitate ointment.
			Erythematous.	Papules may be acuminated or broad. Are first rose colored, surrounded by white border of scales. Later they have a tawny hue. Most marked on the nape of the neck, flexor surface of extremities, perineum and genitals. Appears between third week and fourth month. Lasts from three to eight weeks.	Potas. iod. and Merc. corr. Locally: The 5 per cent. oleate of Mercury.

VI. NEW GROWTHS.	OF GRANULATION TISSUE.	SYPHILIDES.	Vesicular.	May be *herpetic* or *varicellaform*. *Herpetic vesicles*, are millet-seed or pea-sized, and are seated on coffee-colored base. May be arranged in circles or segments of circles. They last a week and disappear without scarring. *Varicellaform* vesicles are about the size of small peas, are surrounded by coppery red areolæ, and are occasionally umbilicated. Form greenish-brown scabs. Leave purplish discolorations. On face mostly. Sixth month after chancre.	Merc. corr. Cinnabar, and Merc. iodide. Locally: Merc. corr. lotion or the Oleate of Mercury.
			Pigmentary.	"Coffee-with-milk" colored macules, varying in size from a cent-piece to a half-dollar. Oftenest in women. Mostly on neck. Lasts one or two months. Comes between fourth and twelfth month.	Nitric acid or Calcium sulphide.
			Pustular.	Three forms: 1st. Millet-seed sized ephemeral dead-grey-colored pustules, which dry and form brownish rough scabs on forehead, angles of mouth and base of nose. 2d. Pin-head or split-pea sized acuminated pustules, which form brownish scabs, and leave small, white depressed cicatrices. On scalp, face and trunk. 3d. Ecthymatous umbilicated pustules. Size, from a pea to a hickory-nut. Have dark areola. Greenish brown scabs, which leave copper-colored cicatrices.	Kali bich. and Merc. nit. Locally: White precipitate ointment.

VI. NEW GROWTHS.	OF GRANULATION TISSUE.	SYPHILIDES.	Bullous.	Pea to walnut-sized blebs. Dark, greenish-brown scabs. Rare. May occur in the newly-born.	Potass. iodide. and Syphilinum.
			Squamous.	Small red circular blotches covered with scales. Leave dark colored spots. Commonly symmetrical. Sixth month after chancre.	Merc. precip. ruber. Arsenicum sulphide. Cinnabar. Sarsaparilla. Merc. corr. Phytolacca, etc. Locally: Red precipitate oint.
			Tubercular.	Circumscribed dome-shaped brownish-red elevations. Split-pea or walnut-sized. On face and back. Leave pigmented spots brownish or blackish scabs covering punched-out-looking ulcers. Figure-of-eight appearance of eruption.	Merc. bijodat. and Potass. iod. Thuja (*mucous tubercles*). Locally: Treat the tubercles with Acid Nitrate of Mercury, and dress the ulcers with Iodide of Starch paste.

VI. NEW GROWTHS.	OF GRANULATION TISSUE.	SYPHILIDES.	Gummatous.	Appears first as hazel-nut sized hard lumps, situated on head, buttocks, and flexor surfaces of the extremities. Either single or multiple. Undergo absorption or break down, and form deeply-excavated ulcers. A tertiary syphilide.	Carbo animalis. Condurango, etc., and remedies for the tubercular. Berberis aqu. Bi-cyanide of Mercury. Cistus for mercurio-syphilitic ulcers.
			In Children.	Decline in health. Fissures and chaps about the mouth, anus and genitals. Skin dry harsh and dingy yellowish hue. Face wrinkled. Looks like little dried up old man. Snuffles. Hoarse cry. Coppery-red mucous patches. Dry or moist papules. Tubercles. Bullous syphilde. Excoriations and mucous patches most common.	Calcium iodide. Corallium rub. Locally: A five per cent Oleate of Mercury inunction.
VII. NEUROSIS.	DERMATALGIA.			An affection of the skin characterized by pain, unattended by structural change. Attacks principally covered parts. More in women than in men. Sensitive to external impressions. Pain worse at night, of a burning, boring, or shooting character. Lasts a week or longer.	Baryta carb. Bell. Bry. China. Ferrum. Manganm. Nux mosch. Phos. Sepia. Silicea. Spigelia. Sul., etc. Galvanic current.

VIII. PARASITIC DISEASES.	VEGETABLE OR DERMATOPHYTIC.	TINEA FAVOSA. (Favus.) (Honey-comb Tetter.)	Characterized by pea-sized, straw-colored, cup-shaped, honey-comb crusts. Stale straw odor. *Achorion Schonleinii.* Contagious. Poorer classes. Mostly on head, frequently on the trunk.	Bromine. Kali carb. Lycop. Mezereum. Phos., etc. Epilation. Parasiticides. Hyposulphite of Soda, Merc. corr., or Sulphurous acid lotion. Chrysophanic or White precipitate cerate.
		TINEA TRICOPHYTINA. (Ringworm.) (Barbers Itch.)	Characterized by itching erythematous redness and crop of vesicles followed by scaly formation. On scalp, hairs become brittle and break off. Stubble-like appearance. On body, spreads in fairy-ring-like manner. On head, split-pea or hazel-nut sized papules or tubercles appear. Hairs come out without pain. On nails, called *Onycho-Mycosis.* Follicles occasionally, pour out viscid mucus resembling juice of the mistletoe-berry (Kerion). Contagious. Children of lymphatic temperament. *Tricophyton.* In youth attacks scalp or body. In adult life the beard. Fungus scales or scabs turn whitish yellow on addition of Chloroform.	Sepia and Tellurium (*Ringworm*). Merc. precip. ruber. Kali bich. Plantago. Tart. emet. and Cicuta (*Barber's Itch*). Cocculus Indicus, etc. Epilation. Shaving every other day. Merc. corr. or Sulphurous acid lotion. Acetic acid or Coster's paint. Chrysophanic Cerate or White precipitate oint.

VIII. PARASITIC DISEASES.	VEGETABLE OR DERMATOPHYTIC.	TINEA VERSICOLOR. (Variegated dandruff.)	Fawn-colored patches accompanied by itching and desquamation. In phthisical patients between ages of twenty and forty. Chest and abdomen. *Mapped appearance. Microsporon furfur.* Next to tricophyton in frequency. Feebly contagious.	Sepia and Natrum ars. Mild parasiticides. Sulphurous acid lotion. Acetic acid baths.
		ALOPECIA AREATA.	Characterized by more or less sudden appearance of variously sized white bald patches. Starts on parietal protuberances. Frequently unilateral. Oval areas devoid of hair. Spreads rapidly. *Smooth polished surface.* Fine lanugo.	Phos. Natrum mur. Fluoric acid. Calcium sulphide. Mancinella. Phos. acid, etc. Epilation of marginal hairs. Acetic acid, tinc. of Arnica, Cantharis, or Capsicum applications. Merc. cor. or weak Phosphorus lotion.

VIII. PARASITIC DISEASES.	ANIMAL OR DERMATOZOIC.	GUINEA-WORM DISEASE.	Due to the *filaria medinensis*. Common in tropical climates. Pointed tumors surmounted by blebs. Swelling and pain. Tumor breaks, and shows the worm.	Remove the worm. Dress sore, as a common ulcer.
		ELEPHANTIASIS. (Elephant leg.)	Due to the *filaria sanguinis*. See class IV.	
		MITE DISEASE.	Due to the *leptus irritans*. "*jigger*." Papules, vesicles and pustules. On ankles and legs. South-western states. Along the Mississippi. Mostly in summer.	Mild parasiticides. Sulphur ointment.
		PHTHIRIASIS. (Lice disease.)	Due to pediculi. Contagious. Three varieties: P. capitis, P. corporis, and P. pubis. *P. capitis*. Occipital region. "Nits" in children. "Scratch marks." *P. corporis*. Ova or pediculi deposited in clothing. Multiform lesions. On trunk, hips and thighs. "Scratch marks." *P. pubis*. Due to crab louse. In adults mostly.	Oleander *P. capitis*) and Mercurious. Locally: Powdered Staphysagria. Cocculus ind. tinct., White percipitate oint., Merc. corr. lotion or Chloroform application. Bake the clothing.

VIII. PARASITIC DISEASES.	ANIMAL OR DERMATOZOIC.	SCABIES. (Itch.)	Contagious disease due to the *acarus scabiei*. Characterized by cuniculi attended by *nightly itching*, and formation of papules vesicles and crusts. Occurs mostly in the interdigits and on wrists, in flexures of body, buttocks and dorsal surface of penis. Seldom above the nipple line. Multiform eruption. Evidences of contagion. Disappears rapid-under parasiticidal treatment.	Sulphur. Locally: Sulphur oint. Storax oint. Oil of lavender. Balsam of Peru, etc. Bake clothing.

PART IV.

ORTHOEPIC GLOSSARY.

Ac'a-rus (*acarus*, mite). A genus of minute insects infecting the skin.

Ac'a-rus sca-bi-e'i. The itch insect.

Ac'ne (*acme* top). *See* Part II.

A-cu'min-at'ed (*acumen*, a point). Pointed.

Ag'ri-us (*agrios*, fierce). An adjective signifying inflamed.

Al-o-pe'ci-a. Baldness.

Al-o-pe'ci-a a-re-at'a. *See* Part II.

An-æ'mi-a. Deficiency of blood.

An-æs-the'sia. Loss of sensibility.

An-i-dro'sis. *See* Part II.

An'-thrax (*anthrax*, a burning coal). *See* Part II.

A'-rea. An open place.

At'ro-phy. Deficient nutrition.

At'ro-phy, lin'e-ar. *See* Part II.

Ax-il'læ. Arm-pits.

Bac-chi'-a. A synonym of Rosacea.

Bleb. A synonym of Bulla.

BROM-I-DRO′-SIS (*bromos*, a stench). Fetid perspiration.

BUL′LA. A water-bubble. *See* Part II.

CA-CHEC′TIC (*kakos*, bad). Pertaining to a depraved condition of system.

CAL-LOS′I-TAS. *See* Part II.

CAN′CER (*a crab*). *See* Part II.

CAR′BUN-CLE (dim. of *carbo*, coal). A synonym of anthrax.

CAR′RON OIL. A mixture of about equal parts of lime solution and flaxseed oil.

CHAUL-MOO′GRA OIL. Expressed from the seeds of the Gynocardia odorata.

CHIL′BLAIN. A synonym of Pernio.

CHLO-AS′-MA. *See* Part II.

CHLO RO′-SIS (*chloros*, green). Green sickness.

CHRO-MI-DRO′-SIS (*chroma*, color). *See* Part II.

CI-CA′TRIX. A scar.

CIN′-GULUM (a girdle). A synonym of Zoster.

CLA′VUS (a nail). *See* Part II.

COM′E-DO (a glutton). *See* Part II.

CON-DY-LO′MA-TA (*kondulos*, a tubercle). *See* Part II.

CONI′DIA. Fungus spores.

CRUS′TA LAC′TEA (milk crust). A term formerly used to designate Eczema of the face in children.

CU-NIC′ULUS (a burrow). Made by the itch insect.

CU-RET′TE. A small scoop.

CYST (*kustis*, a sac). *See* Part II.

DAN′DRUFF. Scurfiness.

DE-PIL′A-TO-RY. A remedy which causes the hair to fall off.

DER-MA-TAL'GI-A (*derma*, skin, and *algos*, pain). *See* Part II.

DER-MA-TI'TIS. Inflammation of the skin.

DER-MA-TI'TIS CON-TU'SI-FORMIS. *See* Part II.

DER-MA-TI'TIS EX-FO'LI-A-TIVA. *See* Part II.

DER-MA-TOL'O-GY (*derma*, skin and *logos*, discourse). That branch of science which treats of the physiology and pathology of the skin.

DER-MA-TO-LY'SIS. *See* Part II.

DER-MA-TO-PHY'TON (*derma*, skin, *phuton* plant). A vegetable parasite.

DER-MA-TO-ZO'A (*derma*, skin, and *zoon*, an animal). Animal parasites.

DER'MOID. Resembling the skin.

DYS-IDRO'SIS (*dus*, difficult and *hydros*, sweat). *See* Part II.

EC-THY'MA. *See* Part II.

EC'ZE-MA (to boil up). *See* Part II.

ELE-PHAN-TI'A-SIS (*elephas*, an elephant). *See* Part II.

EM'BO-LISM. Obstruction of a vessel by a clot.

EN-DEM'IC. Belonging to a particular district.

EPH'E-LIS (*epi*, upon, and *helios*, the sun). *See* Part II.

E-PHEM'E-RAL. Short lived.

EP-I-DEM'IC. Generally prevailing.

EPI-THELI-O'MA. *See* Part II.

ER-Y-SIP'E-LAS. *See* Part II.

ER-Y-THE'MA (*eruthaino*, to redden). *See* Part II.

FA'VUS (a honey-comb). A synonym of Tinea favosa.

FI'BRO-MA (*fibra*, a fibre). *See* Part II.

FI-LA'RI-A MED-I-NEN'SIS. The Guinea-worm.

FI-LA'RI-A SAN'GUI-NIS. An animal parasite; the cause of Elephantiasis.

FIS'SURE (*fissura*, cleft). *See* Part I.

FRAMBŒ'SIA, pronounced *fram-be'she-a*, from *framboise* a raspberry. *See* Part II.

FUN'GUS (*fungus*, a mushroom).

FUR-FUR-A'CEOUS. Scaly.

FU'-RUNC-LE (*furunculus*. a petty thief). *See* Part II.

GRAN'ULE. A little grain.

HAUS'TEL-LUM. A sucker.

HER'PES (*herpo*, to creep). *See* Part II.

HIR-SU'TIES. Hir-su'she-es, (*hirsutus*, hairy). *See* Part II.

HY'-DRO-A (*hudcr*, water). *See* Part II.

HY-'DRO AD-EN-I'TIS. *See* Part II.

HY-PER-Æ'MIA. Excess of blood in any part.

HY-PER-ÆS-THE'SIA. Over-sensitiveness of the skin.

HY-PER-IDRO'SIS (*huper*, in excess, and *hidrosis*, sweating.) *See* Part II.

HY-PER-PLA'SIA. Excessive formation of tissue.

HY-PER'TRO-PHY. Thickening or enlargement.

ICH-THY-O'SIS (*ichthua*, the scale of a fish). *See* Part II.

IM-PE-TI'GO CON-TAGIO'SA. *See* Part II.

IN-CRUS-TA'TION. The act of forming crusts.

IN-DU-RA'TION. The process of hardening.

IN-NER-VA'TION. The act of giving nervous energy.

IN-TER-TRI'GO (*inter*, between, and *tero*, to rub.) *See* Part II.

KE'-LOID. *Kele*, a crab's claw. *See* Part II.

KE'-RION (*kerion*, a honey comb). A term formerly applied to

SU-DAM'I-NA (*sudo*, to sweat). *See* Part II.

SY-CO'SIS (*sukon*, a fig). *See* Part II.

SYPH'I-LIDE. *See* Part II.

SY-PHIL'I-DES. Skin diseases arising from syphilis. *See* Part II.

TE-LAN-GI-EC'TA-SIS. *See* Part II.

TIN'E-A. A moth-worm. *See* Part II.

TIN'E-A FA'VOSA. *See* Part II.

TIN'E-A TRICH-O-PHY-TI'NA. *See* Part II.

TIN'E-A VER'SI-COLOR. *See* Part II.

TRI-CHI'A-SIS. *See* Part II.

TRICH-O-CLA'SIS. *See* Part II.

TRICH-O-PHY'TON (*thrix*, hair, and *phuton*, plant). The fungus of tinea tricophytina.

TROPH'IC (*trophe*, nourishment.)

TU'BER-CLE (dim. of *tuber*, a swelling). *See* Sec. 2., Part I.

UM-BIL'I-CATED (*umbilicus*, the navel). Depressed in the center.

UR-TI-CA'RI-A (*urtica*, a nettle). *See* Part II.

VAR-I-CEL'LA-FORM. Resembling varicella.

VIS'CID (*viscum*, bird-lime), gluey, adhesive.

VER-RU'CA. *See* Part II.

VES'I-CLE (dim. of *vesica*, a bladder). *See* Sec. 2, Part I.

WHEAL, pronounced "*hweel.*" *See* Sec. 2, Part I.

XAN-THO'MA (*xanthos*, yellow). *See* Part II.

XER-O-DER'MA (*Xeros*, dry). *See* Part II.

ZOS'TER (*zoster*, a belt). *See* part II.

PART V.

METRIC TABLE.

APPROXIMATE WEIGHTS.

1 Milligram	=	0.015 gr.
1 Centigram	=	0.154 gr.
1 Decigram	=	1. 543 grs.
1 Gram	=	**15.432 grs.**
4 Grams	=	1 fl. drachm.
1 Kilogram	=	2½ lbs. avoir.

APPROXIMATE MEASURES OF LENGTH.

1 Millimeter	=	0.039 in.
1 Centimeter	=	0.394 in.
1 Decimeter	=	3.937 inches.
1 Meter	=	**39.37**

The United States "nickel" five-cent piece weighs five grams, and is two centimeters in diameter. (Haines.)

A meter is about the one ten-millionth part of the earth's polar quadrant.

APPROXIMATE FLUID MEASURES.

1 Cubic Centimeter	=	15 minims	=	¼ fl. drachm.
4 Cubic Centimeters	=	**60 minims**	=	**1 fl. drachm.**
1 Liter	=	15,000 minims	=	**1 Quart**

An ordinary back-gammon die is about the size of a cubic centimeter. (Haines.)

PART VI.

BIBLIOGRAPHY.

ALLEN, T. F. Encyclopædia of Pure Materia Medica. 10 vols. New York.

ANDERSON, M'CALL. Treatment of Diseases of the Skin, with an Analysis of Eleven Thousand Consecutive Cases. London. 1872.

BÆHR, B. Therapeutics. 2 vols. New York. 1875.

BULKLEY, L. D. Eczema and its management. New York. 1881.

—— Manual of Diseases of the skin. New York. 1882.

BUMSTEAD. The Pathology and Treatment of Venereal Diseases. Fourth edition. Philadelphia. 1879.

COWPERTHWAITE, A. C. Elementary Text-Book of Materia Medica. Chicago. 1883.

DAMON. The Structural Lesions of the Skin. Illustrated. Philadelphia. 1869.

DUHRING, L. A. A Practical Treatise on Diseases of the Skin. Philadelphia. 1882.

FOX, TILBURY. Skin Diseases. Second American, from third London edition. New York. 1875.

FOX. Epitome of Skin Diseases. Second American edition. Philadelphia, 1879.

FRANKLIN, E. C. A Manual of Venereal Diseases. 1882.

HEBRA (& KAPOSI). On Diseases of the Skin, including the Exanthemata. New Sydenham Society. Translation.

HEITZMANN. Microscopical Morphology of the Animal Body. New York. 1883.

HILLIER, THOMAS. Handbook of Skin Diseases. Philadelphia. 1865.

HOYNE, T. S. Venereal and Urinary Diseases. Chicago. 1883

HUGHES. Therapeutics. London. 1877.

JAHR, G. H. G. Diseases of the Skin. Edited by Hempel. New York. 1850.

—— Forty Years' Practice. New York. 1869.

—— Venereal Diseases. New York. 1868.

KAPOSI. Pathologie und Therapie der Hautkrankheiten. Wien und Leipzig. 1882.

LILIENTHAL, S. Diseases of the Skin. New York. 1876.

—— Homœopathic Therapeutics. Second Edition. New York. 1879.

LIVEING. Hand-Book of the Diagnosis of Skin Diseases. New York. 1879.

MEGNIN, P. Les Parasites et les Maladies Parasitaires. Paris. 1880.

MORRIS, MALCOM. Skin Diseases. Philadelphia. 1880.

NEUMANN, ISIDOR. Hand-Book of Skin Diseases. Translated. New York. 1872.

PIFFARD, H. G. An Elementary Treatise on Diseases of the Skin. 1876.

—— A Treatise on the Materia Medica and Therapeutics of the Skin. New York. 1881.

RUSSELL, J. R. The Skin and its Diseases.

RAYER, P. A Theoretical and Practical Treatise on Diseases of the Skin, with colored plates. From Second London Edition. Philadelphia. 1845.

RAUE, C. G. Pathology, and Therapeutics. Philadelphia. 1882.

—— Annual Record of Homœopathic Literature for 1871-2-3-4-5. New York.

RUDDOCK, E. H. Text-Book of Modern Medicine and Surgery on Homœopathic Principles. London. 1874.

VANBUREN & KEYES. A Practical Treatise on Surgical Diseases of Genito-Urinary Organs, including Syphilis. New York. 1875.

WILLAN & BATEMAN. A Practical Synopsis of Cutaneous Diseases. Philadelphia. 1818.

WILSON, ERASMUS. On Diseases of the Skin. A System of Cutaneous Medicine. Sixth Edition. London. 1868.

YELDHAM, S. Homœopathy in Venereal Diseases.

INDEX.